I dedicate this book to Lucy.

This book is about my experience in the NHS as a student nurse from 2011 to 2014. All the names of the patients I cared for, and the staff I worked with, have been anonymized to maintain confidentiality.

Contents

Chapter 1: A new Career

I had enjoyed being a performer my entire life, I attended a three-year drama degree in London, and took part in many plays, and after graduation I managed to gain the lead role in Peter Pan, traveling all over the country. However, my whole world was turned upside down when I received a phone call from my identical twin brother Michael in our hometown of Yorkshire.

I remember that day so clearly, I hurriedly bought a ticket from Marylebone station in London back to my hometown. As I arrived home, my brother was sitting on his bed in the room we shared. I sat next to him, he explained he had been diagnosed with brain glioblastoma grade four. He had developed a serious malignant brain tumour and had to leave his job as a doctor. Michael's form of cancer was the most advanced form of brain cancer, in which the survival rates of patients is only between 12-18 months.

I broke down in tears that day, I was devastated, I couldn't imagine a life without my brother. That summer, we spent three months doing all the things we always wanted to do. We travelled to London, and went on the open-top bus tour, taking in all of the London sites, we travelled to Cornwall and learned how to surf, and then we went to a publisher, who had approved of Michael's comic book templates, a dream of his was accomplished to get his comics published.

It was then in late July that I came across a poster 'Become a nurse in Yorkshire and change lives.' Something struck me about the poster, now that my brother was suffering from a terminal illness, and I had taken time out of my acting work, I wanted to help others. I secretly applied for the adult nursing course, passed the interview, and waited to start on the course the following September.

Chapter 2: First Placement

I remember the first day I arrived at the hospital. It was a beautiful bright Monday morning. As I stood on top of the hill, outside the hospital, in North England, I gazed in awe at the three-story hospital building. I had left my job as a successful actor in London to train for a job, I had always admired. I had spent five years caring for my elderly grandparents at the weekends, my favourite television show was casualty, and surely training as a student nurse was the right path for me?

I slowly walked into the huge hospital, as I entered the revolving doors I was faced with big escalators and three lifts. I wore my long white student nurse jacket, hidden by my long green army-style coat, and my blue striped trousers. I could feel my heart racing, I was feeling both fear and excitement. I was about to start my first student placement on the General medical elderly ward.

I walked up to the large green doors and pressed the purple intercom, "Hello its Chris, the student nurse ready to start my first day," I mumbled. "I beg your pardon," reported the angry voice behind the intercom. The doors were suddenly released, and I began to nervously step onto the ward. I looked down the long ward, in shock, the ward had four patient bays, a large circular nurse's station, a staff room, and three patient toilets.

I could hear a range of noises as I walked onto the ward, I could hear Intravenous machines bleeping, call buzzers going off like an enormous horn, and Patients calling for help.

I walked into the staffroom, sitting nervously down in the tiny handover room, surrounded by five nurses, a sister, and four healthcare assistants. I became bewildered as I sat and listened to the nursing handover, I had never come across much of the medical terminology, and I had never interacted with elderly people in a hospital setting before.

When the morning handover ceased, a bubbly young nurse with tanned skin, wild curly hair, and bright blue eyes sat excitedly next to me. "Hello, I'm Helen I'm going to be your mentor," she beamed. I walked around with her as she introduced me around the thirty-five bedded ward, letting me know where the bedpans were kept, the hospital clothes, and toilets. I followed my mentor as she completed her drug round, looking around in awe and fear, at the patients in their beds. Some patients were attached to drips, and many were sleeping, all the men in my bay were over eighty years of age and were suffering from a range of conditions such as diabetes, confusion, and arthritis.

As my mentor completed the drug round, she explained that it was time to complete the patient washes, she pulled the curtains around six of the patients, and gave me a washbowl, with warm water, "here you go, you can wash your patient," she beamed enthusiastically. I walked in and there sat the elderly gentlemen waiting for me to help him with his wash. He sat in his bright orange pyjamas with long grey curly hair. The nurse then threw a towel over the curtain which landed on my head. "Hello, I'm Chris, I've come to help you with your wash this morning," I smiled. The patient then proceeded to remove their trousers and urinated on the floor, "Oh dear," I gasped in shock, as the patient continued to walk around causing a large puddle to form on the floor. I used a towel to soak up the urine and stood in shock. I had never washed a person other than myself before; I was in shock to have to help people with such a range of needs. Some patients required full assistance with washing everywhere whilst others were independent. I felt accomplished when the patients thanked me for my efforts.

It felt strange to finally be on the wards, I had spent over two months at the university on a 'mock ward' putting plasters on ghoulish wide-eyed mannequins, completing first aid training, learning about effective communication, and now I was in the REAL environment. My mentor asked me to make the beds for all of the patients, I mistakenly believed it would be an easy job, until my mentor arrived back from her break, with her mouth open wide, "well at least you tried!" she grimaced, "you've made the beds back to front," giggled the healthcare assistant.

I finally felt like I was completing clinical duties when my mentor asked me to complete nursing observations. I had spent weeks learning about the physiology behind taking measurements for blood pressure, the heart, and temperature, and it felt great to finally be partaking in clinical duties. I happily put the blood pressure cuff on the elderly man, and as his arm started to gently compress, his relatives sat back and observed him. "Arr look at him, looks scared out of wits," laughed the elderly lady, wearing a grey tracksuit, with grey fuzzy hair, and wide-brimmed glasses. "He barely looks old enough to be fit to take a paper round," added her gentlemen friend.

I had to get use quickly to sarcastic comments, I was visibly nervous and had a permanent look of fear on my face, and I looked at all times like 'the new person.'

I went into the sluice, a place where all the dirty linen and toiletries were kept. Inside the room was a macerator, where the cardboard boxes were crushed in and filled with water. I put the ten bowls in the macerator and suddenly a strange rumble came from the machine, and the lid burst open and water spilled all over the floor, seeping out of the room, as the machine exploded with a loud thud. I walked outside the sluice room, to a shocked look on the ward manager's face.

The entire sluice room was covered in shattered broken pieces of the macerator. I became bewildered on my first day on the ward at how much work the nurses had to do, with washing patients, administering medications, answering phone calls, liaising with a wide range of NHS staff, it almost seemed like a juggling act, keeping up with numerous roles and duties.

The visitors came in from 2pm to 4 pm breaking up the peaceful atmosphere. Suddenly a range of visitors came up towards me asking me a range of questions, 'how is my husband?' 'When is my brother coming home?' 'Doctor, can you update me on my Grandad's medical condition?' I felt very overwhelmed, unable to answer the questions. I resorted to sitting down in the spinning chair at the nurse's station feeling hopeless.

Every task I completed seemed much harder than how I imagined, getting some patients out of the beds, required assistance with mobility aids, such as hoists, walking frames and standing aids. I was so inexperienced, I had to have a second member of staff to help me with all tasks. My mentor had drawn up a range of tasks for me to complete, including the care rounds, measuring the catheter urine output, recording the patient's fluid intake, assisting patients to the toilet. I had so many patients and family members ask me 'am I knew?' 'When did you leave school?' I was scared that I wasn't going to make it through the training, the twelve-hour shift was filled with so many tasks and challenges, and I needed help with each one!

At the end of the shift I started to feel dizzy, as I stood by the nurse's station, I felt faint and collapsed onto the chair. My mentor and another nurse came rushing towards me, they took my temperature which was unusually high at 40 degrees. "Go home now, and well done on your first day," she smiled. I went home exhausted, I wondered if nursing really the career choice for me was.

When I arrived home each day, I would spend time with Mum and Michael. Michael spent most of his time during my first placement, in the study continuing his writing pursuits. He was doing everything he could, to keep his mind off his illness. He remained so positive, taking our dog Rex for a walk each morning, and he would go swimming in the local community university gym. Then he would go to volunteer at our local community hospital. I never spoke in great detail about my nursing experience with Michael, after work we would often stay up late to watch scary movies, and listen to our music, we were both

grateful for each day.

Chapter 3: Learning to be a Nurse

I had arrived apprehensively each morning to the shift, knowing as a student that my actions were constantly being watched and scrutinized. I went onto my first night shift, feeling relaxed and calm. The atmosphere was so different at night, staff members were not rushing around, all you could hear were the snores of the patients, and the beeping from the iv machine, as I looked into the bays, the patients looked so peaceful, and relaxed, laying in their beds or so I thought.

An hour into the shift, I heard sudden screams from patients in the bay, along with windows being smashed, I crept nervously down the corridor, as I reached the bay, I witnessed a shocking scene, a confused patient had smashed all the windows in the bay and threw water from the jugs over the sleeping patients. "Sir Calm down," I pleaded, waving my hands to try to evoke a calming reaction. The elderly man stood there by the smashed glass on the floor, looking at me in anger, his face red with frustration, "it's your fault, you sent me into this prison," he shouted. "No, if you come towards me, we can talk about this," I whispered. My calm response worked to no avail, the patient angrily grabbed their walking stick, and charged towards me, I cowered on the floor, before the night sister grabbed the stick saving me!

Eventually, as a team we had to dry and change the wet patients, the confused patient had to be given one to one assistance from then on, and we promised he would escape 'the prison,' eventually.

Whilst working as a student, I quickly realized that the hospital environment was not a conducive environment for confused patients to stay in, with different staff on each shift, different sounds, and new patients each day. it was not a suitable environment in promoting continuity in their lives.

As days passed on the ward, I became more comfortable in my abilities as a

student nurse, whilst still being unable to shake off the image as the 'new guy.'

I still seemed to be attached to my mentor, with most activities such as administering medications and completing dressings, requiring direct supervision. We seemed to have certain patients who stayed on the wards longer than the other patients.

One elderly gentleman would sit in his chair, every day and not move, he was a man who came in from the street, a man who had lived on the streets for over twenty years. He wore a grey dirty suit, which was covered in thick dirt, and left a stale odour. His hair was long and knotted, and his teeth black from poor dental hygiene habits. Each day, I would offer to assist him with a wash, each time he would refuse, he had nowhere to go, but was refusing to improve his physical condition. I watched him sit happily each day, as he tucked into his warm meals, and lay in his comfy warm single bed.

An Elderly gentleman who resided in the side room, would greet me each morning in anger, taking a disliking to me, he would throw items at me such as fruit, his bowl of porridge, and his lemonade bottle. Each morning when he threw items at me, I would have to duck quickly. He came into the hospital with confusion, each time I tried to talk to him, I never seemed to make it through his bedroom door.

A lady who suffered from dementia, and had been on the ward for two months, found life very difficult on the ward, she spent her whole life as a nurse, and believed that she still was. She would walk through the ward in her colourful long ball gowns, and six-inch high heels, with her long hair wrapped up in a bun. Sometimes she would sit at the nurses' desk, sometimes sitting there smiling at the nurses, whilst at other times she would attempt to guide the patients' relatives with their queries.

At times when there were patient notes on the nurse's desk, she would grab a random folder and record in 'her diary'. Sometimes she would refer to herself as 'the sister.' The patient would become increasingly aggressive and fed up with staying on the ward as the day continued, she would run for the main door, and try to escape, and then cry as soon as she was taken back to her chair.

I remember a young patient who had been on the ward since I started my placement, he was twenty-nine years old, he came in diagnosed with type 2 diabetes, and he had difficulty in maintaining stable blood sugars. Throughout his time on the ward, his blood sugars would increasingly become more erratic, until one day I discovered the reason. When he walked to the toilet one afternoon, I found an empty sweet packet on the floor, as I knelt down, I looked under the bed, and underneath were five cardboard boxes, in one box were six bars of dairy milk bars and five cartons of beer.

Suddenly I could hear the Patient shout from behind me, "What are you doing? That's private property!" he shouted. "I'm sorry but you really shouldn't be eating sugary food! It will affect your diabetes!" I warned him. Eventually, after much frustration on his part, he retracted onto his bed. I could feel his glare of anger towards me. I did have to report what I found to my mentor, which had caused the patient to become even more verbally angry towards me. It was then that I realized the significance of my role, I was training not just to help the patients, but to educate them, on how to improve their own personal habits, to protect their own health.

It was with the patient with type 2 diabetes, that I had my first emergency; it was on the final day of my placement that the emergency occurred. I was walking behind my mentor as she completed her drug round, when I looked at the patient in the bed, I instantly became worried, he was sitting up in his bed shivering, his face was pale, and he was mumbling, and when I tried to check if he was alert, his speech became incoherent and slurred. I realized that the patient was having a 'hypo attack,' which occurs when a patient has a blood sugar under 4 mmol/L.

I remembered what my mentor had taught me about treating a hypoglycaemic episode. I rushed over to the treatment room; I could feel my heart pounding, the rush of adrenaline surging through me. I grabbed the blue diabetes treatment box, which contained a fast-acting glucose drink and glucose gel, used to help raise a patient's blood sugar in the event of a 'hypo.' I gave the patient the drink in his hand as he began to shake, helping to hold the drink towards his lips, I then rubbed the glucose gel onto the patient's gums and watched as he regained his composure, and it worked, the patient was able to overcome their hypo attack. It felt wonderful being able to help a person overcome an emergency.

I had learned so much over the course of the placement, communicating with elderly patients, taking observations, and responding to emergencies, but the road to becoming a nurse had only started, I was just at the beginning.

Chapter 4: Respiratory ward

I remember when I started my second placement on the respiratory ward. I had expected a different experience to the other ward, but it was very similar, as most of the patients were admitted with a range of medical conditions, from cancer to ulcerative legs, to patients who were sent in for detox from alcohol addiction. I walked onto the ward at 7am, on a cold November morning, it was a frosty morning and it was pitch black outside.

As I arrived on the ward, all the lights were flashing in the bays, and I could smell the warm cooked breakfast, of bacon and sausages and fresh toast, simmering on the plates. As I walked onto the ward, I could see staff members rushing around, the night staff were rushing out to leave the shift, while the day staff were getting ready for handover. I sat in the handover room surrounded by a mixture of young and newly qualified nurses. It was then that I met my mentor, an older lady in her early 60's, with long curly greasy hair, tanned skin with blue eyes, she wore bright red stick.

"Everyone this is the new student called Chris, say hello to Chris," she mumbled. The night staff then began their handover, the ward contained oncology patients, cardiac patients, and the rest of the word consisted of patients suffering from complications in their diabetes condition.

As I finished the handover, I got ready to start the medication rounds with my mentor. "I expect no silliness on this placement, if you start washing the patients this morning, then maybe you can complete the drug round with me in the afternoon," she snapped. Already I knew this wasn't a good sign, my mentor was asking me to give up a vital learning opportunity in favour of taking up a healthcare support role.

I looked around the bay of six women. As I walked into the bay I was greeted by Mary, a patient who had recently diagnosed with dementia and was found wandering in the street, she was dancing in the middle of the bay, to songs by Doris Day. Mary was 90 years old and wore a bright blue nightgown. She grabbed my hands and we danced together in the middle of the bay. I tried desperately to release my grasp, but she held onto my hands tightly, reluctantly getting me to participate in a waltz dance with her.

"Oh, you know what if I was several months younger, I would marry you, because my husband's dead you see," She laughed. I carefully guided her towards her chair and connected her radio earphones to her radio.

The second patient Sheila was admitted with stage three brain cancer, she was a warm and kind sixty-year-old lady. She wore a white nightgown, her skin was pale, and she had brilliant blue eyes, she wore a bright blonde poorly fitting wig. She sat up in her bed, reading one of the several books she had brought in with her. She was a strong-willed woman, she spoke to me about how difficult the diagnosis was for her and her family, and how she had accepted that she was now at the palliative stage. "I know I have lived my life to the full, and raised three exceptional children, and that they are financially secure, and my religion keeps me positive," She explained to me. I walked over to the next patient who was laying in her bed, her eyes open but almost motionless, her name was Deborah, she was 85, and at the end of her dementia illness, she was no longer able to communicate and mobilize, and could only eat soft soluble food. She was a very slim woman, at only six stone, with long curly black hair, she seemed to sink underneath her large brown double duvet. The next patient, Louise, was a forty-year-old obese woman, at twenty-five stone, who was admitted following a struggle to control her type 1 diabetes condition.

The next patient was an ex-nurse Susan aged eighty, she sat in the chair immaculately dressed in a blue overcoat, her hands were covered with her white silk gloves, her face was pale and her eyes were emerald green, she was brought in by her family worried about her recent confusion culminating in her locking herself in the bathroom for two days. "Can I help you? You're looking at me a bit gormlessly," she murmured. "I'm Chris I'm going to be looking after you today." I smiled. "Well I don't need looking after, go ahead about your business and leave me alone," she scowled.

The final lady in the bay was Kate a 99-year-old lady suffering with progressive dementia. She was brought into hospital, as her daughters struggled to look after her at home, she would sleep on a mattress on the living room floor. She had white bushy grey hair, her eyes were emerald green but bloodshot, and she wore a silk cream nightgown. On the table next to her she had a tissue box filled with random items such as a screwdriver, a pencil crayon, a hairbrush, a mood ring, and three Jaffa cakes and a pocket-size crossword book.

"Harry Harry get me out of her!" she shouted. I walked up to her, "hi Kate I'm Chris I'm looking after you today. "Oh, Harry I am so glad to see you, I've been sent to this awful rotten place, take me home," she shouted.

I gave Sheila, Louise, and Susan towels and washbowls so they could wash independently, I worked alongside the healthcare assistant who helped me to wash Deborah, as she was unable to complete any self-care activities on her own.

I went into Kate's bed space and drew the cubicle curtains to assist her with a wash, she became agitated during the wash, "Oh Harry Harry, take me home" she shouted. Suddenly standing behind me was Mary singing, 'Crazy' by Patsy Kline behind me, "Mary you can't come in here, Kate is having her wash," I began, "Is that your mother? Oh, she is a bonny lady," she added. I guided Mary back towards her chair and continued to assist Kate with her wash.

Kate had been unable to mobilize for over a year, as she had slept on the mattress in her front room for over a year, we used a hoist to help her to mobilize into the chair, "Oh Harry help me, God help me please!" she shouted. We made Kate comfortable in the reclining chair, and eventually she began to relax. As I came out from behind the curtains, Mary appeared, "Can you dance with me again?" She asked. "I'm a little busy Mary, maybe later" I added.

My mentor was a really stubborn woman and forgot my name several times, "How are you doing Michael? I'll be able to catch up with you later at 2pm after my meeting ok!" She explained as she strutted out of the ward, striding her arms like a general soldier. I knew already I was dealing with a difficult nurse, every student nurse's worst nightmare, having a nurse mentor who was too busy to look after you due to her management responsibilities.

There I was, left alone with the bay of six patients I felt nervous and unprepared.

Sheila was so helpful and kind, as she went over to the other patients to talk to them, she danced with Mary and helped to reassure Kate that she was safe in the hospital, as she kept on trying to get her legs out of the bed.

The ward was a forty bedded ward, and each nurse and healthcare assistant were put in charge of their bay. The morning was such a busy time on the ward, which consisted of a medication round, followed by washing patients and a drugs round. Then came the doctor's drug round, I walked around with the consultant Dr. Clarke, as he was joined by his junior doctors as they completed their round. I felt my lips start to quiver, and my whole body began to shake, as he asked me for information regarding the patients, I referred to my handover sheet, and tried hard to relay back information to the doctor but I was a nervous wreck, maybe because I was new and inexperienced. I felt intimidated, as a student nurse I felt that I was constantly walking around with a sign saying, 'new person.'

After the drug round, I was called by one of the other nurses to help with the washes in their bay, as I came out I went back into my bay to a concerned Sheila, "Chris, Mary has just ran out I've tried calling her, but she won't come back." I walked around the bay desperately looking for her, but it looked like she had left the ward, and my mentor has just arrived back, "what's wrong with you? You look like a lost goat!" she grumbled. "It's Mary I can't find her I was called into C bay, but she has absconded." I added.

"Well go and find her then, she's your responsibility" she moaned.

I nervously walked around the hospital looking for her in the corridors, as I went down the ten flight of stairs to the ground floor, I could hear someone singing, 'Start spreading the news, I'm leaving today,' As I walked into the Cafe, there was Mary standing on top of the table, dancing, all the other customer looked on in surprise and shock, as she sang so loudly and with great enthusiasm. Eventually, with the assistance of the manager, we helped Mary to climb down from the table. It was then that she became very angry, throwing plates from the table angrily on the floor, her happy mood suddenly turning to anger, which is common for a patient with dementia.

"I don't want to come back to the ward I want to go home to my mother!" she cried, after twenty minutes she reluctantly agreed to come back to the ward.

When we returned to the ward my mentor decided to help me in redressing Mary's ulcerative leg. First, she helped to wash her leg in honey, before using the non-touch technique to put on the latex gloves before carefully applying the multi-layered dressing, "Hopefully one day Arthur you will be able to do this," She began. "It's Chris," I groaned.

That afternoon before the shift had ended Sheila had called me over, as I walked up towards her bedside, I could see she was uncomfortable in the bed, the tissue in her hand, was now covered in blood, she looked up at me helplessly, "Chris things have gotten worse since I've last seen you, the doctors have the results of my current MRI scan, and my cancer has continued to progress, despite the chemotherapy treatment, they say now it will be a matter of weeks now for me."

She cried, as tears swept from her face. I walked up to her and grabbed her hand, "Don't worry I am here for you," I smiled.

It had now been six months since Michael had been diagnosed with brain cancer, he continued to write in the study during the day, but due to his condition when I came home he would increasingly become very tired and collapse in front of the television when I wanted to see him. Also, I had noticed a change in his moods, which became erratic, he could switch from being happy to angry in minutes, I was always there to support him, but found the increasing change in his condition difficult to deal with, and I struggled to sleep at night.

Chapter 5: Happiness and sorrow

As the time passed my mentors behaviour towards me continued to decline, each day she would become 'too busy' to speak to me, often attending meetings, and being taken away to complete 'management duties.' To resolve the problem to myself, I tended to book my shifts with a buddy mentor, who was a newly qualified nurse from Poland, who taught me so many new nursing skills and procedures.

At the end of the second week Sheila's health continued to decline, she was now moved to the side room, it was the first time I had looked after a dying patient. I walked into the side room at the start of my shift, as she lay in the bed. "Chris, can you please help me with my drink? I'm feeling very weak," I raised her head in the bed and assisted her with her drink. I was so sad, a week ago she was rushing around the ward helping the other women in the bay, now she was bed-bound requiring full care.

"I'm so glad you're here today, do you believe there is life after death?" she asked. "I like to believe that there is something after, yes, it would be awful if our time on earth is all we have."

"I believe when you die that we go up to heaven by stepping up a golden staircase, where you are greeted by gold gates, all our pain, worries and troubles are resolved, and anything we dream can come true, I know my parents will be waiting for me," she added. Sheila's room was now filled with a collage of family photos on the wall. I walked around to have a look at the photos. The pictures showed what an eventful life she had led up to this point. In one photo she stood proudly in her graduation outfit holding her nursing certificate, in another photo she was surrounded by her family outside universal studios, in Florida, and in another photo, she was being presented an award for her novel she wrote, 'dignity in nursing' which sold over a million copies over ten years ago.

Later that afternoon Sheila called for help, "Chris can you help me please, I need the toilet" she requested. I left the room to get a commode for her when I entered the room, it was too late Sheila had suddenly passed away.

I walked over to her bed, and looked at her lying peacefully on the bed, a ray of golden light shone on through the window, lighting up her pale face. It was then that I knew all the suffering had gone from her face, she was now relaxed and looked peaceful, and her hands were no longer clenched in agonizing pain, but fell gently by her side. I felt she was a special person, she spent her whole life caring for other people, and after watching her suffering with her condition for over a month, I knew now that she was finally at peace. I held onto her cold hand as I slowly closed her eyes which were still open.

As a student I had to make the devastating phone call to Sheila's family to tell them that there had been a sudden change in their mother's condition. It was the hospitals policy not to break bad news over the phone.

I remember her daughter's coming into the hospital ward, we had to take them into the meeting room to tell them what had happened. Sheila's daughters were identical twins in their sixties, both wearing long yellow raincoats, with long curly blonde hair, and they both wore dark thick-rimmed glasses.

As they sat down on the couch, the daughter's eyes started to fill up, they started to cry, "She's dead, we know, we could tell by your voice," she cried. The two sisters tried desperately to regain their composure, before handing me a red envelope with my name on the front. "Mum had prepared cards for all of us in the event of her death and she had this card for you, to thank you

for your help." I nervously opened the card,

'Dear Chris,

I want to thank you for all the care you have provided me, you

really have made a difference to my wellbeing since you have arrived on the

ward. You are very kind and compassionate, please stay strong and keep up

the fantastic work, you have truly made a difference to my life,

Best wishes Sheila.

As the daughters left the room, tears started to stream from my face. That

letter of acknowledgment made all the work I completed on the ward

worthwhile, I made a difference to a dying woman's life, and tried to make her

as comfortable as possible. I cried to myself that evening in the staffroom, it hit

me that I would have to go through losing Michael this way. I could not

imagine my life without him.

Chapter 6: Emergency

I remember walking onto the ward halfway through my placement, after spending weeks avoiding my mentor who did not have the time to teach me, I walked into the ward and bumped into her, "where have you been John? We must catch up," she began. "Well I have been working with Nurse Kate, and she has decided to take over duties in being my mentor," I added.

I quickly moved away from the sister, she couldn't even remember my name, I knew she wouldn't care that I switched mentors.

The ward was so busy, it was December, and it had been snowing for over a week across Yorkshire, the ward was filled with people coming in due to trips and falls, and some had simply been admitted, as they were unable to travel to the supermarket in the poor weather conditions to eat an adequate meal.

My new mentor Kate had decided to give me a day of managing my bay on my own. Mary was still on the ward singing and dancing to anyone who would listen. On this particular shift, I was working in a very challenging bay, of six male patients admitted with dementia and confusion, athlete's foot, and one man was at the palliative stage of his condition.

After I completed the medication round with Kate the nurse, I was left in the bay on my own, "You must stay in the bay at all times, Alfred cannot walk on his own and needs observation at all times," She persisted.

As I looked around I could see the difficulties I would face, Albert was an 85-year-old man, who was unable to stand on his own, as he was very unsteady but insisted that he wanted to go to the airport to see his mother. The patient opposite Albert called Clive, who was admitted with confusion, became very angry at me, holding his wooden stick in his hands, threatening to hit me at any point where I came close to his bedside.

At one point he became very angry at my 'stupid smile' he grabbed all the fruit in his bowl, his apples, bananas, and pears and aimed them towards me, hitting me each time. Clive and Arthur had both stayed on the ward for over two months, as their families had been unable to find a suitable nursing home placement for them, which could accommodate their aggressive behaviour.

I struggled to offer the best care I could give to Donald the palliative patient, who required full assistance, as we were so short-staffed on the ward. There was meant to be three nurses and two healthcare assistants on the shift, but two staff members called in sick, which meant that my mentor had to take charge of the ward, and I had to work extra hard. Working in the NHS really is a collaborative partnership, and each team member on a shirt counts in providing the best possible care.

I found it very hard on this shift, at one point when I was providing personal care, for Donald, Clive stood up and started to smash the ward mirror with his stick. Then Albert's safety alarm which made a noise each time he stood up, kept on making a noise, as he repeatedly stood up and down on his chair. I found myself running forwards and back To Donald, Albert, and Clive the entire shift. I truly realized how difficult it was to take charge in a bay, when you have to work with patients with a range of mental and physical difficulties.

I managed to complete all my jobs that day, completing the patient washes, doctors' round, dressings, and referrals which managed to show I was a competent worker on the ward. However, I had never felt so stressed, the patients with dementia required one to one care, and I felt like a clown juggling all my nursing duties while also making sure the patients in my bay were safe and comfortable.

That afternoon my mentor Kate entered the room said that she would take care of the patients in my bay, as she wanted me to go down to the eye theatre to observe a cataracts procedure being completed. It was to be the first time I would observe a procedure in theatre. As I went down with Brenda, the patient, and the porter, I was immediately aware of how cold it was in the theatre. I began to shiver at the sudden drop in temperature.

As the patient lay down on the operating theatre table, the surgeon showed me the operating table, which he had clearly prepared with the medical instruments he needed to undertake a cataracts procedure. The surgeon pointed at the operating table, "you see this it is a sterile field as long as you sit still, and keep away from this table you will be fine," he grumbled, looking at me with his bride bushy eyebrows drowning in his blue operating coat.

As I watched the surgeon inject a needle into the patient's eye, I began to feel dizzy, I felt hot and confused, and so overwhelmed being in the room. It was then that I grabbed all the items on the sterile field, falling onto the tray that held the medical instruments. I had passed out onto the floor. I then woke up, laying on a black hospital trolley in A and E.

As I opened my eyes, standing next to me was my mentor Kate looking down on me with concern. "I hope you are ok Chris you took quite a bump. Do you think you'll be able to continue your shift on the ward?" She asked. "I think I'll manage," I whined. I struggled to complete the rest of the shift I had banged my head on the floor and felt very weak. There was no room for fainting in the NHS, I had to carry on and keep up the hard work hard.

As we walked back onto the respiratory ward, Kate continued to take over the care of the bay, whilst I helped to look after the other patients due to the short staff issues. As I walked further up the ward, it was then that I heard the emergency button siren go off, the red light in the entrance of the women's bay flashed repeatedly. Suddenly, I felt my heart start to pound, as sweat dripped down my face, a surge of adrenaline fired through me, as I ran towards the bay. I grabbed hold of the crash trolley, and walked into the bay where an elderly lady, at 92, was reported in being unresponsive and required emergency CPR. Suddenly, the bed was surrounded by doctors, nurses and physiotherapists, over twenty members of staff from other wards were around the patient, to help in the emergency.

Suddenly the registrar fired instructions to the staff 'get a drip stand' 'start the compressions' 'next person start compressions.' I felt my hands trembling, as I took items out of the emergency trolley, breathing tubes, and oxygen masks to assist in the CPR treatment. I watched, nervously, as the nurses and doctors completed thirty compressions onto the unresponsive patient.

It was now my turn to have a go, I felt my face boil red with pressure; I completed thirty compressions, and breathed air into the pocket face mask. I continued the compressions until I became tired, and a doctor helped take over to complete the compressions. It was then that I noticed the patients eye flicker and they started to breathe. The CPR compressions had worked, and the patient had regained consciousness.

"Well done team, you worked excellently today fantastic work!" beamed the cardiac consultant. I felt after the emergency, that I had really exceeded my own expectations in being able to save another person's life. I walked back into my own bay that afternoon and my mentor looked at me with pride, "you have worked so hard today I'm so pleased with you, do you want to go home an hour early?" she asked. I leaped at the chance of going home early, although I had achieved so much that day, I longed for a warm dinner and a cold drink. I had been so busy all day but was too busy to stop for lunch.

This was what it was like working on the frontline in the NHS, trying to juggle looking after patients, dealing with emergencies, work in conjunction with family members, and write my notes, and be a functioning human being all at the same time.

Chapter 7: The stroke ward

I had now spent six months as a student nurse and had learned so much I had experienced how to look after a patient, how to respond in the event of emergencies, and how to look after the dying patient. I felt like I was really exceeding in my chosen career path.

For the final three months of my placement, my mentor Kate was moved to the stroke ward, and I decided to move to the ward with her, I would try anything to keep away from the dreaded sister on the ward.

The stroke ward was the busiest ward I had worked in, it was a forty-eight bedded ward which consisted of a stroke assessment unit, which was where people who had just been diagnosed with a stroke were sent. Then there was the ward area which contained forty beds, and at the end of the corridor was a large gym rehabilitation centre, were people who had just had their strokes were sent to in order to rehabilitate. Up until now I had spent time on wards which claimed to be a specialty such as 'respiratory' but were wards filled with general medical patients.

My time on the stroke ward was one of the most valuable learning opportunities I could ever gain, knowing how to fully care for a patient, and work in conjunction with physiotherapists and occupational therapists to help patients learn to walk again.

I will never forget the first stroke patient I looked after Steven, he was a forty-year-old man, a high-flying businessman, who had spent over twenty years traveling around the world, with his successful telephone business. He had noticed he was feeling muscle spasms prior to the stroke, then one morning on his way to the airport to Florida, he began to have a stroke, he explained he could feel his speech becoming slurred, he felt dizzy and weak, as he climbed out of his car, he collapsed onto the ground. I remember when he came into hospital, he was bedbound.

He sat in his bed crying, as I helped my mentor to assist him with a full wash, the physiotherapists were only able to complete passive arm and leg movements until he regained muscle control again. As time passed, his speech slowly returned, with speech and language support, and although he required a hoist to help him into the armchair, he started to move his fingers.

I remember after a week off on the ward, and returning to see how depressed he had become, "I never thought this could happen to me, what about my job? What about my girlfriend? I can't live my life being wheelchair-bound for the rest of my life," he cried. Tears of desperation streamed from his pale face.

"You will get your life back again, I have every faith in you," I assured him. As a student nurse, I didn't have all the answers, but I promised to work alongside him, to help improve his condition.

I asked my mentor if I could observe the patient's physiotherapy treatment, and what I witnessed was a radical transformation, each day the patient would progress further through the treatment, the physiotherapist's practiced sit to stands with the patient, and after two days the patient was able to stand unaided. As days went on, the patient practiced mobilizing using the Zimmer frame, taking one to two steps to increase confidence, until after two weeks on the ward the patient was able to use the frame independently. After one month of physiotherapy treatment, the patient practiced walking by just holding onto the physiotherapist's hands, and when the physiotherapists released their hands, the patient was able to walk independently. I watched as tears streamed from his face, "I did it! I did it," he beamed.

The patient had made a remarkable journey from being bed bound to walking unaided.

I remember seeing the patient months later, out shopping with his fiancée having made a recovery, he thanked me for my help but also stated he could not remember much about his stroke rehabilitation program.

I remember an elderly gentlemen Simon who had been brought onto the ward after having a full stroke. He lived in a small flat with his wife and two older sons. A stroke has such a strong effect on the brain, that it affects a person's thinking and spatial awareness, each person on the ward responded to their stroke differently, whilst some patients made a full recovery, other patients were left with a permanent disability. The stroke had affected Simon severely, he was never able to regain his speech, and did not respond to physiotherapy treatment, and was confined to being in a wheelchair despite the stroke team's best effort.

Many patients who came onto the ward were still at work, ranging from jobs such as working as a dentist, an accountant, and even a highly skilled artist. I had worked so hard on the wards for over four months and had learned so much, it was a world away from my previous job as an actor, but I truly enjoyed helping people, despite the challenges I would face on a daily basis.

It was now Christmas day, and I was on annual leave for two months, spending quality time with my Mum and Michael. I felt like my social life had come to halt when I started my nurse training, I was so busy working and supporting Michael in my time off.

On Christmas Eve, we received two visitors, Michael's best friend Ernest who he trained with at Oxford, and his fiancée Emily. I watched as they both came into the dining room, they both wore wooly coats. Ernest was six-foot-tall, tanned, with wild blonde curly hair; Emily was five foot six, with pale skin, and long wavy brown hair. They both sat down with Michael at the kitchen table. "Why didn't you tell anyone about your illness? Why did you walk off the ward? We could have helped you! You need your friends!" Ernest stammered. "I didn't want to burden you, it's hard enough going through this illness, we looked after dying patients, and treated patients with cancer on the wards, I never thought I'd be facing death at twenty-four," he cried.

It was then that Emily reached into her satchel, and showed a present she had for Michael, wrapped in golden wrapping paper with a red ribbon. Michael opened the present, and uncovered an invitation to be their best man, and a six-week scan of their baby with a note attached, requesting him to be Godfather.

Michael stormed up the stairs and locked himself in his room. It all became too much for him, he was upset that he would never be able to get married or become a father, the reality of his illness set upon him.

In the New Year, in January, I planned a trip to Alnwick with Michael. We lived in Alnwick when we were children, and I thought it was the perfect place to raise his spirits. Michael fell asleep for the entire journey. When we arrived, we slowly walked up the beautiful scenic country roads, to Alnwick Castle. We gazed into the distance, at the beautiful snow-covered mountains. Alnwick Castle is where the Harry Potter films were made, when we arrived, we toured the castle, threw snowball's at each other, and enjoyed the magic show.

We spent the afternoon on Foxton beach, the beach we enjoyed as children, next to the cabin where our Grandparents lived. We sat on the rocky hill watching the sunset. We must have sat for an hour in silence, all we could hear were the crashing of the waves against the sea, the wind blowing the sand, and the seagulls flying above us. I looked at Michael and for the first time in months, he looked happy and content. "We need to talk about the future, about when I'm gone," he pleaded. "No, we have to keep positive, this is not the time for that!" I persisted. "I just want you to be happy, I know you're enjoying the nursing course, but you were an amazing actor. You need to do what makes you happy, you were born to be on the stage," he added.

We sat contently watching the sun go down, before walking to the hotel and finally going to sleep.

For the next few days, we had a great holiday, we raced each other at the go-karting centre, we went skydiving, and swimming in Foxton beach, and we had dinner at Michael's favourite restaurant, Cafe rouge every day. On our last day, we had our lunch on the beach, and played badminton, before getting an elderly couple to take our picture. When we reached the train station, Michael hugged me, "thank you for a great trip, I've had such a great time, it's been the perfect goodbye to my favourite city," he smiled. "Yes, I wouldn't have missed it for the world." I said, taking a deep breath, before I started to cry.

Chapter 8: Community nursing adventures

After completing my time in the ward, I was sent back to university for two months, to undertake the theory side of the course. I had to complete two exams, including performing health assessments on mannequins, matched to real-life hospital scenarios. However, I strongly believed the only place where you could learn to be a nurse would be carrying out the job by completing practical placements.

Two months after I finished my block period of university study. I received my allocation for my third placement, at a Yorkshire community service, which helped to prevent hospital admissions, through patient assessment and treating patients at home.

When I arrived at the community nursing building, situated in a small Yorkshire village, I was prepared with my fob watch, notebook, and coloured pens. When I walked into the building and into the nursing office, already I was met with great differences compared to the ward setting.

All the nurses were sitting down at their desks, with computers in rows on ten. The room was divided into two, one half of the room was the district nurses, who visited patient's homes each day to complete nursing duties. The other team was 'the community stay at home service' who I would be working with over the next two months. The team included two nurses, a matron, a physiotherapist, and a doctor. My mentor was Hayley a nurse in her forties who had been a nurse for over twenty years. June was a sixty-five-year-old nurse with over forty years of experience, whilst Brenda was a newly qualified nurse with over two years of experience. "Hello, I'm Chris I start a placement here today," I beamed. They ushered me to an empty desk, asking me to put my belongings in the drawer underneath the desk area.

"You're very welcome to the team; we are a hospital at home service we work to keep patients out of the hospital, by supporting them in their own homes following discharge. Your hours of work will be from 9-4 pm each day. We will be out all day say you will need a nice warm coat," She smiled.

Already as I sat at the desk, I felt a sense of calmness, gone was the chaotic environment of the ward, in which the nurses were constantly juggling many jobs at once. Working with the community nurses left me feeling calm, relaxed, and content.

That morning I was to spend the morning with June, the most experienced nurse on the community team. She was a wild character, she was five foot one, with long curly blonde hair, tanned skin, she wore a bright purple dress and had a white cardigan draped over her shoulders. I hopped into her yellow small Peugeot, as I got in, she smiled at me, "you don't mind cigarettes, do you?" she asked. "No," I lied, I hated cigarettes and coughed continuously throughout the journey. I could not prepare myself for June's atrocious driving, she would often hit the pavement, and narrowly missed two bikers and cars on the road. I wondered how I would ever get through the days shift, as we had a caseload of fifteen patients to see, but we we're getting nowhere fast.

We reached a derelict country road, surrounded by beautiful golden crop fields. Suddenly Nurse June let out a wild scream, "Fucking hell, where did they come from?" She screamed. I peered out of the window in shock, suddenly, we were surrounded by a herd of cows blocking our entry. "Get the bastards away go out and distract them," she requested. This was not how I envisioned my first day on my community placement. I climbed slowly out of the car trying desperately to shoo the cows away, and then I fell onto the muddy ground, all of a sudden, my perfect white uniform was ruined, black and mud stained. I stepped back into the car as the cows slowly moved away, "A bit of dirt never hurt anyone," June laughed giggling at me.

We carried on down the narrow road until we reached our first patient's house. The first lady that we went to see was a seventy-year-old lady who lived alone in her four-bedroom bungalow. She had recently been discharged from the cardiac ward at the local hospital but was struggling at home. As we knocked on the door, we waited five minutes but there was still no answer. We saw an elderly lady peering through the net curtains. She opened the door, "I'm sorry I didn't answer I thought you were a pair of Mormons," She laughed.

We slowly entered the door, and we looked around in surprise, all the walls were covered in pictures of bulldogs. "I've been really struggling since leaving the hospital, I try to complete my housework, but I become very breathless most of the time. We sat down on her leather couch and measured her oxygen saturations, her poor reading meant that she would now require oxygen at home. The patient was suffering from COPD chronic obstructive pulmonary disease, which was linked to years of smoking, and she was now at the beginning of her heart failure condition. I could see already how valuable the community service was, if the patient had just been left at home on her own following discharge, concerns such as her breathlessness on exertion would not have been raised. June showed her pictures in a booklet of oxygen machines that she could have specially fitted into her house.

"I do feel quite lonely being stuck at home all the time, my children have all moved on now, and they both live abroad, I don't really have anyone to speak to." she sighed, looking out of the frosted window. "Well we can offer you a buddy system, we can send a hospital visit to your house once a week, to take you to the hairdressers or to the local communication centre," she assured her.

"You have a lovely house, have you ever owned one of these bulldogs?" I asked, pointing at the endless pictures of the dogs on her walls. "Oh, you haven't met Trixie!" she beamed, walking slowly up to the garden door, releasing Trixie into the house. Trixie was a large aggressive black bulldog, she scurried into the house jumping excitedly onto June, before turning around and snarling her teeth at me, before pouncing on me. I held onto her face as she desperately tried to snap at me with her large teeth. "Oh, dear she's usually such a mild-mannered dog!" she warned, managing to carefully pull the dog away from me. "Just go in the car," June warned. I had just visited my first patient and was almost killed! It was one of the many events which showed me that you cannot predict what will happen when you enter a patient's house.

We then proceeded onto the next patient's home; June talked me through her own nursing journey. June trained as a nurse in the 1970's and worked as a nurse auxiliary for two years from the age of seventeen, almost all of her training took place on the ward, and she only spent a number of days in the classroom. Nurse training had shifted now towards more academic work, in where written work holds equal importance to practical nurse training in the ward.

It was then that June helped me to prepare for my next visit. We arrived in a rundown area in Yorkshire to a private street. As we stepped out of the car June pulled a box out of the boot of her car, filled with latex gloves and plastic bags. "We need to wear these gloves and put the bags over our feet for the next patient's house," she warned. "Mr. Topping has recently been discharged from hospital, he has been living alone for the past thirty years since the death

of his twin brother, and he is struggling with his alcohol addiction." She began.

"Why the gloves and bags?" I asked. "Well his house is a little unkempt and

dirty, it's just to keep us away from infection" she added.

As we walked towards Mr. Toppings house, we realized that the door was left

open, suddenly an angry looking woman appeared from next door, in her

white dressing gown with short curly black hair, "if you're looking for Mr.

Topping you won't find him yet, he goes walkabout, and returns about 1 pm in

the afternoc n, God knows where he goes, I just wish he went for a bloody

wash he stinks," she yelled. It was then that we made the slow walk into Mr.

Topping's house.

"James are you upstairs?" June called out but there was no answer. We stood

in shock in the living room, with the bags over our feet and gloves on our

hands. The curtains were drawn, there were unopened letters all over the

floor, the green couch was covered in piles of blankets, as I lifted them up a

tower of dust filled the air nearly choking me.

In the dining room, pictures of clowns hung all over the room, June Explained that Mr. Topping was the ringmaster for the traveling circus in the 1940's. The room had a strong musty smell, a strong smell of faces and the room smelt as if a dying wild animal has inhabited the house. "What we will do is, we will quickly look around the house, and leave, this is obviously not a habitable environment," June warned. Adjacent to the dining room was Mr. Toppings Kitchen, which was both small and basic, having just a round wooden table and a fridge. The floors were filthy and covered in faeces and food droppings, the cooker was deeply rotten, and in the frying pan were piles of bread which were deep green with mould, and flies swarming around them. June opened the fridge and let out a sigh in desperation, all the food in the fridge was covered in green mould and covered in cobwebs. The house looked like a scene from a horror film.

We slowly crept up the narrow wooden staircase, to check the rooms upstairs. Upstairs, the bedroom was filled with piles of clothes dumped on top of each other, piles of books were left cluttered together, pictures of clowns and a picture young Mr. Topping as the ringmaster of the circus hung on the hallway wall. We entered a closed bedroom door, and all of a sudden June let out a terrifying scream, "There's someone in the bed!" she shuddered, she believed she had seen someone, and ran around the stairs in a great panic, I followed behind her. Then Mr. Topping entered through the front door. He wore a dirty grey suit, with a blue flat cap, carrying a large bag of potatoes. He collapsed onto the pile of mud ridden blankets on the sofa.

"You know we can really help you with your house, we can get a cleaner in to help make sure the house is clean, we can also send someone to help you with the shopping," June smiled. Mr. Topping became very angry and began to wave his walking stick at the both of us, "Get out my house you patronizing pair of gits," he shouted, grabbing me by the shoulder. We quickly hurried out of the house, and June explained that all we can do is refer what we seen to the social services and contact his next of kin," she explained.

I felt so sad for Mr. Topping, we struggled to stay ten minutes in his home, it was as if he had just given up on his life, I wanted to help him but couldn't at that point.

We travelled further through the village that morning until we reached a suburban village and entered the next home of our patient Margaret. Margaret had recently been diagnosed with dementia and was referred our service by her daughter, who was worried that her mother's memory was deteriorating, reporting that she had left the cooker on all night, and had difficulties completing self-care tasks on her own. Margaret's daughter had taken a trip to America for two weeks, so she wanted the team to check on her.

We knocked on the door, and Margaret rushed to the front door, she stood in her green suit, black wavy hair and thick black glasses "Oh quick come in my favourite film is on!" she beamed.

As we walked in, we could hear the musical Annie on full blast in the living room, she slipped into the room, singing 'the sun will come out tomorrow' She asked us to sit down. As we walked into the kitchen, we could see worrying signs that she wasn't coping, the cooker was left on, and she had bowls in the kitchen filled with breadcrumbs with no other food in the fridge. As we sat down we noticed Margaret had red blotches all over her face arms and legs, it turned out that she was having an anaphylactic shock, her face and lips started to slowly swell, and June injected her with a needle to give her adrenaline, and she was put on oxygen, whilst I called the ambulance.

The ambulance arrived and she was finally taken to the hospital, as she was taken in, she struggled to recall basic facts, such as her age, address, and names of her children, which showed impairment in memory and a fast decline in her cognition.

A few weeks after going into hospital and after talking to her daughter Margaret agreed that she could not cope in the house on her own and was sent to an assisted living accommodation with care assistants.

It was only my first day and already an emergency occurred. We carried on in June's car to the other patient's houses. We arrived at a forty-year-old single lady's house. Her name was Lucy, she was diagnosed as clinically obese, being over twenty-five stone, and was also clinically depressed. Lucy was part of the community service for treatment of her chronic leg ulcers and needed her insulin injection each morning for her diabetes condition. As we entered the house, I looked on in shock as in every corner of the house were stacks of magazines in every room including, 'hello' and 'ok' magazines. Lucy was resting on her king size sofa bed which was situated in the living room.

I took her blood sugar reading, which was 16 mmols, way over the normal blood sugar of 4 moles. Under her sofa chair she had chocolate boxes, sweets and crisps underneath the chair, "you really are going to have to cut out all the sugar and fatty foods, your blood sugars are still going to be erratic, and greatly affect you," June warned. "It's not easy here, I live alone, my husband left me and has taken the kids," she sighed. "Have you spoken to your GP who can get you in touch with a counselling service? June asked. Then Lucy began to cry hysterically, "I do need help, but I can't do it on my own," she pleaded. That meeting with me and June on that day proved pivotal to Lucy as that week she accessed the help she needed by visiting her GP and getting the counselling help she needed. Lucy managed to lose six stone in a year, and after gastric band surgery, she managed to return to work as a customer assistant at the local supermarket.

As we returned to the office at 3 pm, we were both so tired, although it was still so early in the day, if we were on a ward, we would still have over four hours left of our shift. So much had happened, and I was exhausted from the day's events. We arrived back at the community office and completed our notes on the computer.

My time in the community setting offered me valuable experience as a student nurse, getting to see the other side of nursing, by seeing how patients manage at home, and just how difficult life can be for elderly people, and how a range of factors such as loneliness, depression, and weight problems can affect a person's health. Over the coming weeks, I went to a range of different patient's house, some days there would be no answer at the doors, sometimes my mentor would stay and seem to talk about her whole life history, I was always on hand to take the patients observations, the heart rate, and blood pressure check. I had learned more hands-on nursing skills on the wards but felt like going into community helped me to see a different side to nursing and helped me to improve my communication skills.

For the final few weeks of my placement, I spent some time at a local GP clinic assisting the doctors and nursing with the dementia screening support program. The clinic which specialized in dementia diagnosis, supported patients and families from initial diagnosis of dementia to treatment at home or hospital, for patients with the late stages of dementia. I remember the first patient I seen in the clinic, a 50-year-old lady, she had asked for her clinic sessions to be recorded, to help aid her with her memory.

The doctor showed me a clip of her first meeting, she had long blond curly hair, bright blue eyes, and wore a green overcoat and wide brimmed hat. She was on leave for her job as lawyer, due to her deteriorating memory problems. In the video the doctor asked her a range of screening questions, 'I want you to remember this address 38 Wood Green street, East London, we will come back to it later' 'I want you to spell green backwards", he then proceeded to show pictures of different farmyard animals, and asked about her deteriorating memory.

She was unable to recall the name of the street earlier in the interview and she was unable to recall the name of certain farmyard animals. The doctor requested that she would undergo a CAT scan to check for changes in function of the brain. "I'm really scared Doctor, for the past five months, I've been forgetting work appointments, I can't sleep at night, I'm really worried," signed the patient. The patient then expressed then expressed how she had worries of being diagnosed with Alzheimer's disease as her mother died from the condition at 70 years of age.

When she came into the clinic, it had been exactly a month since her first visit, the doctor asked her husband how she had been over the previous month. "We've really struggled as a family, she barely sleeps at night and wondered around the house, she forget her way to work last week, and asked for directions, she's also had trouble in remembering her brother's name when he visited last week," he said, worriedly.

The doctor looked at both the patient and her husband with a glum expression, taking off his glasses. "There is no easy way to say this, but I've looked at your CT scan results, and I can confirm you are suffering from early onset dementia, in this case Lewy body dementia. I watched as she sat looking on helplessly as she stood up,

"This can't be true, my mother went through this, her condition progressed so fast that she was unable to care for herself and was sent to a nursing home!" she screamed, walking out of the clinic. "How can she have Alzheimer's disease at fifty, well I want a second opinion, we'll go to a private hospital, how will we cope? "What will we tell the kids?" gasped the husband, holding his head in his hands, crying in desperation.

It was shocking to see the effect a diagnosis of dementia could have on people, early onset dementia is rare, and this poor woman was on the brink of losing her job she worked so hard for, due to the shocking side effects of this fast progressing disease.

Over the next few weeks at the Doctors clinic, I met many different patients diagnosed with dementia. As the days passed, I wondered how cruel the condition of dementia was, making people forget essential parts of their lives, forget their family members and eventually forgetting who they are.

It had now been over two years since Michael's diagnosis, he would spend almost half of the day sleeping in his bedroom, he struggled in completing personal care tasks, and required assistance from care assistants, and used a walking frame to help with his decreasing mobility. I remember one evening going upstairs and I could hear him crying, he was throwing items angrily around the room. I sat next to him and hugged him wondering why he was so upset. "Why has this happened to me? I'm only 24 I really wanted to continue my career as a doctor, to have a family, now I have nothing" he cried. As I

hugged Michael, I took a deep breath, I couldn't allow myself to be upset, I had

to stay strong for both of us.

My time in the community settings seemed a longer period than the time I

spent on the hospital wards, due to the wards being 'pressure cooker'

environments, in which there were tasks to be completed each minute. I

continued to have more adventures with June, such as being locked in a

psychiatric patient's house in the evening service, her car breaking down and

spending the day walking from house to house. We also got locked in the lift at

the community base for over five hours, were June repeatedly swore the entire

time.

Over the six-week period in the community setting, my routine seemed to be

similar each day. We went to the nursing home firstly each morning to

administer insulin injections to the elderly patients. We would then visit

patient's houses to complete dressings, take observations and offer health

promotion. At 3pm each day we returned to the office to complete our nursing

notes.

Through my community placement I got to spend more time with Michael at home as we finished at 4pm each day. The weekend before the end of my community placement, I was awoken by Michael coughing in the middle of the night uncontrollably. As I rushed over to him, I realized he had been coughing blood. I went with Mum and Michael to the hospital, and we waited in the A and E department all night, the scan results had shown that Michael's cancer had spread, he had been offered a stronger form of treatment, but Michael refused based on the strong side effects of the treatment.

On the Sunday it was our 25th Birthday, Mum had decorated the house in blue and red balloons, and bought us a five tier birthday cake, Michael spent most of the day in bed, whilst I sat in the dining room watching the home alone films, anything to keep my mind off the inevitable fact, that this would be our final birthday together.

As night approached, Mum had invited people to our party, my old college friends, and Michael's past hospital colleagues. Michael even managed to come downstairs to interact with everyone, until my Dad showed up out of the blue. He arrived at the doorstep with his satchel and presents for us, looking scruffy in blue dungarees, with his long grey messy hair and scraggly beard. Dad had walked out on us over five years ago, Mum and Dad's relationship fell apart. He nervously walked into the room, "Chris, Michael, we need to talk, I found out last week about Mikes' illness." Suddenly Michael ran past us in a rage, grabbing my Mum's keys to her range rover, and sped off down the road. I followed in my car, whilst Mum and Dad argued on the doorstep.

Michael continued to drive faster down the long narrow road through the fog, until he reached the mountain area, I got out of the car and chased him through the forest area to the mountain top. Michael stood at the edge of the cliff, "Don't come any closer, I'll jump," he shouted. "No, you can't! You can't leave me like this!" I pleaded. Then mum and Dad who followed behind us ran towards Michael, hugging him, Dad and Michael broke down in tears, "I'm so sorry, I'm sorry for everything'." Dad Cried.

Chapter 9: summer job

In the months following the community placement, I gained employment in hospital and community settings, through my University employment service. I worked on different medical and surgical wards, and worked alongside the nurses in community settings, including clinics and going out to patient's homes.

I completed my first shift at the hospital's sleep physiology ward, which is a booked in service in where patients suffering from sleep disorders are sent to, and stay on the ward overnight, and their sleeping pattern is monitored, and the report is sent to the specialist sleep physiologists. I entered the office at 11pm at night, and sitting at the desk was a healthcare assistant, "who are you? What are you doing here? I usually work here alone!" Snapped the care assistant, in her white cloak and dark curly hair. "I'm Chris, I'm here to help". Then the care assistant showed me the large television on the screen on the wall, it showed the patient sleeping, it showed the patient's vital signs, including their heart rate and breathing rate which was consistently recorded. The patent had been suffering from narcolepsy, a brain disorder which causes people to suddenly fall asleep at inappropriate times and needed to be monitored.

As I sat, desperately trying to keep awake monitoring the screen, the care assistant brought in a large picnic bag, and took out a wide selection of foods, spring rolls, chicken wings, a dozen sandwiches, and a large chocolate gateau cake. Then she sat at the desk putting up her feet, before watching her favourite film 'beaches' on her phone, "oh you don't mind, do you? I like to have a snack and relax a while at the start of the shift," She smiled.

I could not believe she could eat so unhealthily, and eat so much, not to mention whilst being on shift! As I monitored the patient on the large screen, I went over to her array of food, I went to taste one of the spring rolls and suddenly the healthcare assistant smacked my hand. It was then that the patient pressed the buzzer to go to the toilet, I went to assist the patient who was attached to multiple coloured wires.

The healthcare assistant then requested that I go to the cupboard to get a new observation sheet. I walked out and looked for the room, I opened one door, turned the light on, and as I walked in the door closed tight behind me. I had entered the waste disposal room; a tiny room were the rubbish was kept. Then to my horror, I attempted to open the door, but I was locked in. I started to panic, I could not stand enclosed spaces, and I began to bang on the door repeatedly but there was no answer. I spent five hours in the room that night, the healthcare assistant opened the door at 6am and stated, "You should have knocked the door and shouted!"

My eyes were really opened to what life was like for nurses on my night shift at a busy A and E department. As I entered at 7pm all the nurses and doctors were crowding around a large circular desk in the middle room. The staff were writing in the notes, talking on the phone, and handing over to the night staff.

All the small cubicles around the desk, were filled with patients and their nervous family members. Suddenly, the paramedics came in pushing in a patient on a hospital trolley, the patient was a twenty-three-year-old man, who had been taken in after a drunken fall from his flat window. Suddenly, staff congregated round him, sliding him onto the hospital bed. Nurses quickly compressed the blood pouring from his head with padded dressings, whilst the doctor took his blood pressure, his heart rate was over 120 beats per minute, and his breathing rate had rapidly increased, as his eyes started to flicker.

It was then the doctor requested for him to be sent to the theatre imminently to help compress the bleeding and prevent haemorrhaging. Suddenly the man's mother, entered the ward, a woman in her 50's wearing a long green coat and red boots, "what happened? Is he going to be ok? He left me an answerphone message, saying he couldn't cope at work, and the only way he could escape would be to commit suicide," she began. It was then that I ushered her to the empty cubicle, as her hands began to tremble, I made her a warm drink.

I then continued to walk around the A and E department, and I helped a young woman who had been stung by a bee, and developed an anaphylactic reaction, by helping to put the prescribed cream on her affected areas. I could see her face and arms were covered in red blotches, and her lips were swollen, and her eyes were red. "I'm lucky in a way, I was sitting outside on the bench of the hospital, on my lunch break, I work in the office block opposite, and I was eating my sandwich when suddenly the bee stung my lips. They said if I had been at work, I wouldn't have made it." She beamed.

It was then that I noticed a young nurse looking frustrated, sitting at the desk with tears in her eyes, "two nurses have called in sick, I have two patients who need bloods taken, but I've only just qualified, and I have a confused patient over there who needs looking after." she sighed. I attempted to help her by assisting the confused patient who sat angrily and agitated in the bed. He sat in the hospital gown, with wide red glasses and grey curly hair. His wife sat next to him in the cubicle, I don't know what to do? I just don't know if he's having a breakdown. This afternoon he picked me up from town, and then we reached a roundabout, but he kept going around for thirty minutes he would exit. The police came, and he managed to stop. I think it must be stress, he works as an accountant, and is up all night, I think it's catching up on him," She said worriedly. Whilst we were talking, we had not noticed that her husband had taken her car keys and exited the ward.

As I walked around the ward, so many different events were happening simultaneously. Some patients were angrily calling out for their discharge medication, some staff were helping to calm down a wounded lady from a road traffic accident, buzzers were constantly ringing, and multiple trolleys filled the corridor, and entrance of the A and E department. It was then that I could see how stressful nursing was, and how unpredictable life was in the A and E department

Chapter 10: Theatre Nightmare

I had enjoyed my time in the community caring for the patients in their homes,

but I was ready now to go back to the wards and future develops my nursing skills. I went back to university for another month of block theory study, before being given my allocation for my next placement.

I was based in a busy theatre in the city centre of Yorkshire, specializing in cosmetic surgery, orthopaedic surgery and cardiac surgery. When I entered the theatre, I was joined by a fellow student Kayleigh, and we were not prepared for who we were about to meet. We entered a large staff room with a round table surrounded by wooden chairs. Then our mentor entered the staff room, she stood in her white nursing dress, she was a large built woman and her belt across her chest look fit to burst, she had a pale face with short blond hair and dark green eyes. "You have to be a very good student to pass with me she!" she warned. She introduced herself as Sister Tracey, and she moved around us to inspect our uniform.

Most of our time in theatre was spent observing the surgery and follow patients from the theatre to the ward to observe the whole surgical journey. In my time in theatre I witnessed patients having knee surgery, facelifts, gastric bands inserted, and various cardiac surgeries. I worked alongside Kayleigh in the recovery area, taking the patients observations, offering a drink after surgery, and then transferring the patients back to the surgical ward.

Our mentor was a tough nurse who liked to belittle and bully students at any opportunity, constantly testing both of us by asking us complex medical questions and asking us to complete drug calculations without the aid of a calculator. I spent every morning, in the staff room with Kayleigh going through common medical terminology, as we were constantly tested, and we felt as if we were on a community service programme rather than a training course. We struggled through, but we made it through to the end of the theatre placement. I had since heard on returning to the wards, that the same nurse had intimidated other nurses on their learning journey, and her deeply disturbing bullying behaviour stayed with me to this today.

 Nursing is difficult and at times a very stressful job which is exacerbated by a bullying nurse.

Chapter 11: The final wish

I was ecstatic to leave the theatre placement and was now ready to enter my final nursing placement in a general medical ward in a small village in Yorkshire. I walked onto the busy ward and was again greeted with patients admitted with a range of conditions from dementia, confusion, gastric problems to heart disease. My mentor was a 37-year-old nurse, from Africa with over fifteen years' experience as a nurse, specializing in cardiac medicine. I felt pressure now as I was entering my final placement as a student nurse and had to really develop and show what I had learnt from my training.

The ward had a welcoming ethos as soon as you entered through the door, nurses and healthcare assistants were always at hand to help you.

I remember my first shift were my mentor asked me to oversee the bay for the day, and she would act as the healthcare assistant. I had six complex patients to look after that day. I had to look after two men in a side room; one man had terminal pancreatic cancer, and had his own room, with a view to a beautiful grand oak tree and park out of the window. My patient in the next room had deterioration in his dementia diagnosis, after smashing all the windows in his house and throwing his television out of the window.

Then I had a bay of patients including a twenty-four-year-old woman who was waiting to be discharged following her knee surgery, the next patient was a lady, aged eight five who had been admitted with confusion. The next patient was a fifty-year-old lady admitted with breathlessness, and adjacent to her was a ninety-year-old lady who had been admitted after being found wandering in the street.

I had delegated the washes for my mentor and assigned healthcare assistant, and I had a list of jobs to complete including, discharges, catheter care, carrying on the admission of the lady brought in with confusion. I felt I was doing a great job, by 10am all the patients were washed, my drug round was completed, and I was about to start the doctor's round.

We completed a ward huddle, in which we would sit in the ward manager's office and have a piece of toast and cup of tea and discuss any updates on the patients in our bays. It was a great time to relax, and rest. Then suddenly I heard a shout, "Quick she's gone!" shouted the porter. I jumped out of the office, "your patient in your bay has just run out of the ward," he warned. I realized straight away it was my confused patient, I ran quickly down the hospital stairs and through the long corridor, I caught a glimpse of the patient running through the corridor. She ran towards the street and walked onto the road, causing the cars to suddenly halt, and was seconds away from being hit by a lorry. "Mrs. Smith you have to come back to the ward please you can't stay here!" I warned. She then proceeded to lie in the middle of the road, as the cars continued to beep their horns. "Please leave me here I just want to go home!" she cried. Luckily the ambulance team arrived to put the patient on a stretcher, taking her back to the ward, were she was given one to one supervision by the mental health nurse.

I continued my nursing rounds as my mentor had updated me about the doctor's ward rounds. My patient in the side room with progressive dementia was supported by the ward dementia activity team. They offered the patient paper and colouring pens, sensory items to touch and feel, old photographs, to help the patient to reminisce, and music which helped the patient remain calm and relaxed. I felt this was revolutionary, as on other wards I had worked on, staff seemed to struggle with looking after patients with dementia, but the activities team, worked to meet the patient's specific needs.

During my shift I was met with lots of questions the young lady who had knee surgery kept asking 'how much longer will it be before I receive my tablets?' Whilst the lady with breathlessness asked, 'when will I see the consultant?' questions I did not have an immediate answer to. As I completed the leg dressing of the 90-year-old lady, I could hear he emergency buzzer ring, it was for my palliative care patient in the side room, a volunteer worker mistaking thought he had gone into cardiac arrest. I went in and he had passed away peacefully in his room surrounded by his family, his daughters and grandchildren. As I continued through the shift, I managed to discharge my young patient who had knee surgery, whilst my patient who came in with breathlessness had to be transferred to the respiratory ward for specialist care. I was so tired having been awake since 5am, I had been unable to take my lunch that morning as I was too busy carrying out my nursing duties.

At 4pm I received a phone call I was dreading; my brother Michael had been admitted onto the accident and emergency ward that afternoon after collapsing in the local shopping centre.

My mentor excused me from the ward, and as I walked towards his room, my mother was sat outside crying, "He's gone, he's at peace now," she grimaced. I walked into the side room in the A and E department, and there was my brother, my best friend, finally at peace in the bed with hands across his chest. I held onto his freezing hand and said goodbye.

I sat next to him for five minutes resting my head onto the bed, I knew this day would come one day, but I knew I would never be ready to let go. After ten minutes the nurse came in, she gave me a hug before passing me an envelope, "I want to give you this, Michael had this envelope with him when he collapsed, it was found in his bag and I thought you ought to see it."

I found my hands trembling as I opened the letter, my mother entered and held onto my hand, he had secretly booked me tickets for my birthday for a trip to New York, to attend the audition of my dreams as the scarecrow for the

'Wizard of Oz' production. This was the audition I had been waiting for all my life, it was our favourite film, and he had passed my resume onto the casting directors who were interested in meeting with me.

Inside the envelope was a note from Michael saying, 'Go for it follow your dream.' This was Michael's final wish for me I knew I had to listen to him.

A month later I arrived at Birmingham airport ready to take my journey to New York. I was days away from completing my nursing career, I had enjoyed my rollercoaster journey as a student, caring for others, saving people's lives, working with other doctors and nurses and making a difference. However, being an actor was where my heart lay, and I boarded the plane and took a deep breath, I was ready to start my new life and follow my dream.

Chapter 12: The history of nursing

Key facts in nursing:

Key facts in nursing:

Between the 1st to 14th centuries, nursing care was given by unskilled men and women, from the 14th to the 17th century the world was faced with plagues and unsafe conditions.

In the 18th century, advancements in nursing included bed warmers, herbal remedies and heat pads.

General Washington wanted women to serve in the revolutionary war to help the wounded soldiers.

In the 20th century Nurse Education was made more prominent by figures such as Hampton Robb and Mary Adelaide Nutting.

Florence Nightingale opened her first school of Nursing, and nursing schools rapidly grew throughout the 20th century.

Nursing has greatly changed throughout history. In the Middle Ages nursing was based upon religion. Many nurses were of nuns or Monks. Hospitals looked after refugees and the typical sick and injured. In the 10th and 11th centuries, monasteries housed hospitals in their premises. Inside the monasteries Nurses were instructed to meet the needs of all patients. Each church was instructed to have a hospital attached to its institution.

In the 1000's Charitable houses were introduced and were vastly different to the care people received in monasteries and churches. Nurses provided richer customers with alms and medicines.

Florence Nightingale brought great innovation to the Nursing profession. In the 1900's Nurses were greatly needed dew to the development of the civil war.

In the 1850's Florence Nightingale helped to care for wounded soldiers in the 1850's. Many soldiers died at the time due to infections from their wounds, and poor hygiene also contributed to the huge fatalities. Nightingale requested from the government for better hygiene facilities in the hospital and battleground. Nightingale and a team of nurses scrubbed the walls of Barracks hospitals, and opened the windows to encourage ventilation, and clean food was given. All these mechanisms lead to a drop in the death rates after this. Florence Nightingale was known in the 19th century as 'the lady with the lamp,' who walked around with a lamp, caring for the sick and injured on her nightly rounds around the hospital. Florence Nightingale revolutionized nursing care, as up until this point, nursing took place in people's homes.

Florence Nightingale opened the first nursing schools in London 'The Florence Nightingale School for Nurses.'

The national diploma in nursing was introduced in 1922. The First World War gave a huge focus to nursing at the time, although many nurses in the war were untrained and left once the war ceased. Following the Crimean War, Queen Victoria, of England, ordered the creation of military hospitals in the 1860's, such as the Royal Victoria Hospital.

Many Nurses in Britain were able to travel with the soldiers during the war and could raise their rank to Brigadier.

Following World War 1 and World War 2, the government put millions of dollars into the healthcare sector, leading to better training for nurses. Some schools ran courses for registered nurses, and developed doctorates and master's in nursing. Nursing has moved far from nurses being doctor's assistants, to participating in clinical nursing procedures, and prescribing medications. From the 20th century nursing expanded into different fields, such as paediatric, orthopaedic, and Neonatal nursing.

Geriatric nursing is a fast-growing area of nursing. As care of those aged over 65, has increased due to people living longer. Care for elderly patients takes place in many settings such as GP surgeries, nursing homes, and assisted living facilities. Nurses improve patients' lives through referring patients to mental health services, managing medications, and reducing issues such as falls and

infections.

Part 2: The secret diary of a student nurse - My Brothers Wish

I dedicate this book to Michael

Contents

Chapter 1: The first wish

I was so nervous about completing my audition for the role of scarecrow for 'the wizard of oz.' production. I remember standing on the stage looking out at the large auditorium, the empty chairs, and the four judges sitting together on the front row, with the spotlight shining on me. A young woman Teresa was auditioning for the role of Dorothy. I looked out at the judges, three men in suits, and an angry-looking woman dressed in a white gown.

We had to recite the scene from 'the wizard of oz.' when Dorothy met the Scarecrow, and I had to recite the signs of the song 'if I only had a brain.' I gave the best performance I could possibly give, at the end of the audition, the judges all looked the same, sitting down, emotionless, glaring at me before the female judge shouted 'next.'

That was it, my audition was over for my dream role, now I just had to wait. I left the auditorium with nervous anticipation, I hoped I did justice for Michael and made him proud. I spent the afternoon walking along the streets of Manhattan, I just had the audition of a lifetime, but I was still mourning the loss of my brother. We had always planned to go to New York and travel together, we had so much planned, but my brother's illness tore our dreams apart. I believed my brother's present for me to travel to New York for the audition, was my brother's final wish, but even though my brother was gone, I was yet to discover he had put plans in place for me to cope with his passing.

I had a coffee inside a small Manhattan restaurant, my head was filled with mixed thoughts. I looked at my mobile and glaring from the phone were over fifty notifications, a dozen missed phone calls from my mother, my placement team, and text message from friends, saying they were 'sorry for my loss.' I had to turn the phone off, I wanted to escape, I could not decide if I wanted to return to the placement setting yet, I knew in my heart I should try and finish it.

I spent two more days in New York, I received a notification that day that I would need to wait over a week for the outcome of my audition. I spent most of my time in the hotel room, with the curtains drawn, on my own in my grief, occasionally frequenting the streets of Manhattan for fresh air. At night I walked through the quiet streets of New York, watching people ice skating on the ice rink.

I arrived home on a hot August morning, I was exhausted after a long eleven-hour flight. I arrived home at 5 pm, mum was laying on the sofa, with the lamp on sleeping. Mum's face was pale, red, and blotchy and she looked as if she had been crying for hours.

As I walked up the staircase and into my bedroom I shared with Michael, his bed was untouched, the imprint from his head was still visible on the pillow. I then looked in the drawers of my desk and found six letters addressed to me, with dates of when they were to be opened. Michael had left six letters, six wishes to help me following his passing.

I opened the envelope, which was numbered one, and inside the note stated, 'to look under the bed.' I nervously looked under Michael's bed where he kept his music records, and then I noticed a present wrapped in golden wrapping paper, I carefully opened it. Michael had created a scrapbook, a collection of all the pictures which captured our childhood. The pictures included our first birthday party at the age of five, at a miniature circus, a picture of us at our high school prom standing with our parents, whilst other pictures included us on a plane preparing to skydive for our twenty-first birthday. Underneath the scrapbook was another present. Michael had copied notes from my diary as a student nurse and compiled them into a laminated scrapbook.

I sat on my bed, that night looking at the entries Michael placed in my scrapbook, trying to decide if I wanted to complete my nurse training.

Chapter 2: The Night Shift

I had been in the medical ward on my placement for over one week, and I was about to complete my first night shift as a student nurse. My mentor Tracey had young children, so she only completed day shifts.

I sat nervously at the nurse's station at 7pm, surrounded by the nurses and healthcare assistants who were on the night shift. I was working with Teresa a thirty-nine-year-old Nurse, from Canada, with over seventeen years of experience, the other nurse was Adel, a fifty-five-year-old nurse who trained as a nurse in the Philippines, with over thirty years' experience as a senior nurse. The healthcare assistants Tracey and Geena had both worked on the ward for over ten years.

After the handover, I went into my bay of four patients to introduce myself. Sheila was in the first bed, an eighty-five-year-old lady who had been admitted with a viral bug, she sat in her bed in her white gown with her sick bowl held closely next to her.

In the next bed was Anita an eighty-six-year-old lady admitted with recent confusion, her family was struggling to look after, and she was brought into the hospital after being found wandering on the streets. She sat in her blue armchair in her bright red dress, she was five-foot-tall and had curly brown hair, and her large brown glasses covered her whole face. Anita appeared happy and content in the chair.

In the opposite bed was Sheila a ninety-five-year-old lady who was admitted with terminal lung cancer and lay sleeping in the bed. The patient in the next bed was Hayley, a fifty-five-year-old lady admitted following a fall, provoked from her excessive alcohol drinking.

I went around with Teresa completing the medication round, and then made sure the patients in the bay were comfortable. With the healthcare assistant, I helped to reposition Shelia in the bed and helped her change into her nightclothes. Hayley was able to take care of her needs independently on the ward. I had to provide Shelly with a towel and a sick bowl in the event of more vomiting episodes.

I went over to help Anita into the bed. "Oh, you are kind, what's your name?" "Chris." "That's a lovely name, oh you are kind helping me into the bed," she smiled.

Anita lay comfortably in the bed, pulling the warm blue sheet over her body, before giving me a warm reassuring smile.

I then proceeded to collect the nursing bed notes and sat by the nurse's station. I cast my gaze over the ward, it was such a quiet environment in contrast to the noisy environment present during a day shift. The nurses were relaxed completing their clinical duties, there was time to sit down for a cup of tea, time to breathe!

The nurse supervising me on the night shift, Teresa, advised me to get a chair and sit at the entrance of the bay, as the women in my bay were of a high risk of falling and required supervision. I sat on the chair and suddenly a light flickered in the bay, Anita had turned on her bedside lamp, and had thrown all her bedsheets on the floor.

I walked over to her, "Who are you! Go away," she shouted. "I'm Chris, I looked after you earlier," "Bastard that's what you are, a bastard," she screeched. I slowly walked away from her, whilst Teresa advised me to remain close in the bay. I continued to go through the care rounds, and complete my notes in the patient's folder, and as I looked over to Anita's bed space I witnessed that she was gone, she was now sitting next to Hayley, who was resting, stroking her hair slowly. I moved slowly towards the bed space, "Can you move her away from me?" asked a concerned Hayley. "Anita can you kindly leave Hayley to rest, it's very late please returns to your bed space," I requested.

"Please piss off! How many times do I have to tell you keep away from me!" Anita shouted, before grabbing a tray of biscuits and throwing them at me. Anita was filled with rage, and then held a bottle of Robinsons juice in her hand, "Anita please put the bottle down," I pleaded. I half expected her to throw the bottle at me, instead, she proceeded to open the bottle and pour the juice over the floor.

Finally, Teresa decided to help me and grabbed a mop and towels to help soak the juice. The senior nurse Adel walked in, "Please Anita can you return to your bed space you are disturbing the other patients," she warned. "Go away from me your ugly fat cow, I don't talk to fat people," she scowled. Teresa and Adele proceeded to stand either side of Anita, placing the Zimmer frame in front of her, she stood up and went to hit Adel who managed to duck, before throwing herself on the floor, rolling around in anger.

It was now as a team, that we started to panic, the other nurses had to stop their duties to assist me and Teresa with the aggressive patient. The other patients in the bay complained that they were unable to sleep due to the high level of noise in the ward. We tried to usher Anita into standing but she refused, we carefully moved tables and chairs back, as she began to reach for items to use to attack us. "You're all a bunch of ugly circus freaks! I've never seen such a room full of ugly people." she growled.

It was then that we had to call security, to help to encourage Anita back to bed. The female security officer Deborah arrived on the ward, in her yellow uniform, "oh look here comes PC plod, I don't follow orders from gormless people like you, so leave me alone!" she shouted.

"You are disturbing the other patients, and if you continue to attack the other staff members, we will call the police," warned the security guard. "Call them see if I care your fat bitch!" she shouted. Anita continued to roll around the floor, whilst the other staff looked on helplessly me and Teresa completed the care rounds of our other patient.

Anita's aggressive behavior had disrupted the clinical tasks of all the other staff, and the ward did not have the provision to employ a mental health nurse to supervise her.

Teresa decided then to send me on my break, I hoped that over my one hour and a half break, that Anita's behavior would have changed. I felt extremely tired during my break, sitting down in the library seemed to exacerbate my tiredness, as I began to write in my placement book, trying desperately to stay awake.

I came back to the ward after my break, and to my surprise, Anita managed to remain calm, as she lay in the bed in her new bed space in the side room. "Anita walked to the side room herself, but she will need you to watch her," Teresa began. I pulled up a chair outside of the room, and saw that Anita was sleeping, a half an hour later, she proceeded to throw her jug of water onto the floor, and threw her sheets onto the floor, constantly calling me a 'bastard.' This proceeded for three hours until at six am the elderly patient Maureen walked over to me, "I couldn't sleep with all the shouting and swearing, do you want me to talk to her?" she asked, "well."

Then Maureen walked up to an agitated Anita who was sitting in her chair, and turned the radio on, the song 'raining in my heart' by Buddy Holly started to play. Suddenly Anita shot me a wide grin, as she listened to the music. "I was a sister on a geriatric ward for over thirty years, we believed music really helped our patients who were confused." she began.

It was then that I learned how quickly a patient's mood can change on the ward, Anita had been agitated the whole night, but listening to the music helped her to reminisce and relax. Maureen and Anita even began to dance together in the room. Sometimes even the simplest of solutions that are right in front of us, can help improve our patient's wellbeing. One thing was for sure

I was exhausted! What a night shift!

I walked downstairs on my first night back from New York and was shocked as I

peered through the gap in the living room door Dad was sitting next to Mum

on the couch both consoling each other in their grief. I decided to leave them alone, before going upstairs to open envelope number two, inside were two keys to a new polo car, the message read, 'I bought this car a few months before my diagnosis now I want you to have it.'

Chapter 3: The Stroke ward

I continued to reflect on my nurse training journey and remembered a shift on the stroke ward, a shift that helped me see how much of a struggle life can be patients at home, and how loneliness and depression were common themes, in the lives of patients I cared for.

I was now on my second placement and had the increasing responsibility that a student nurse faces as they progress on their course. I was not as attached to my mentor as I had been on my first placement and would undertake self-care tasks and clinical observations without assistance.

I always admired the attitude and work ethic of the staff on the stroke ward. Each morning we would complete a multidisciplinary team meeting at 9 am, which consisted of nurses, doctors, physiotherapists, and occupational therapists. One of the consultant's Dr Shrek, was known for coming in wearing strange items of clothes, once wearing a leather dress with platform heels, another time she wore a biker jacket covered in badges and shiny silver trousers with trainers. Today she shocked everyone coming in wearing a striped suit! We waited each morning with nervous anticipation as to what she was wearing. In this meeting, the conditions and treatment of all the patients were discussed. Today it was my turn to handover the treatment of the patients in my bay. I felt incredibly nervous with all eyes on me, and I had sticky post-it notes in my pocket to help me to remember key information. I managed to recall information and treatment plans for the patients in my care.

I made my way into my bay and greeted the patients, I was looking after five female patients, and two male patients in the side room. The first patient was Alana a seventy-year-old patient admitted after an alert from her neighbour, who she invited over, and admitted to them that she was struggling at home. Alana's neighbor called the ambulance as she was worried about the burns on her arm that were clearly untreated.

The patient in the second bed was Katherine a nighty-year-old lady admitted following difficult breathing at home, Katherine lay with an oxygen mask attached to her. The third patient was Louise, a fifty-year-old woman, who at twenty stone was struggling with her type 2 diabetes condition after a collapse at home.

The fourth patient Hannah was twenty-one and had the curtains shut, Hannah was diagnosed as autistic, and was admitted following a self-harm attempt, as she had locked herself in her room for several days and refused to eat.

The fifth patient Sheila was admitted with new onset of confusion and was found wandering in the streets. At one hundred years old, Sheila was the oldest patient I had looked after. The two men in the side room were waiting to be discharged, Clive an eighty-year-old man admitted with diarrhea and vomiting, and Sean a forty-year-old man, admitted with untreated chronic leg ulcers.

Today was a new experience for me a student, as I was shadowing the ward's occupational therapist Catherine, who was to complete three washing and dressing assessments on the patients, and later we were making a site visit to Alana's house, to see if she would be safe upon discharge, or if she would require adjustments.

It was quite a difficult shift, as not only did I need to shadow, but I also had to work alongside my mentor to support my patients. Catherine entered the bay in her green uniform, she had long blonde curly hair, green eyes, and wore thick black glasses. "Good morning folks!" she beamed to the sleepy patients, opening the curtains to let the bright sunshine through. "Right Chris we can complete our washing and dressing assessments now, please get all the washbowls ready for me" she began. We then proceeded to complete a wash and dressing assessment with Sheila. We helped her remove her nightdress, so she could begin to wash her arms, Sheila shot down an angry expression, "What's wrong with you dear?" she asked. "Nothing wrong, I'm just here to assist you if you need help," Catherine smiled. "Come here dear, I want to whisper something to you," Sheila began.

Catherine knelt, and to her shock, Sheila grabbed her head and forcefully soaked it in the bowl of water, "serves you right for staring at me Mrs. Piggy," Sheila snapped. It was then that Catherine asked the health care assistant to complete the wash, as Sheila became very aggressive.

We then carried on an assessment of our next patient Alana who was struggling at home. Alana lay in her bed in a blue tracksuit; she wore dark sunglasses and had short blond hair. She sat crying on the bed. "What's wrong?" asked a concerned Catherine. "Everything is wrong! My husband passed away five years ago, I have no one to speak to all day, and I feel so alone." she cried. We then proceeded to assist Alana with her wash, she had worn her tracksuit jacket for over a month, covering the burns on her arm, and she had bruises on her back and legs from recurrent falls at homes. "Alana do you mind if we make a visit to your home this afternoon. We want to see how we can improve things for you at home." Catherine smiled. "That's fine making sure you check on my cats too," she requested.

I carried on with my duties that day, before my visit with Catherine to Alana's home. Shortly after the washes were completed, I noticed Katherine was struggling more with her breathing, I called the doctor who increased her oxygen level, Katherine held onto my hand, "Don't go, stay and chat with me," she smiled. I held onto her hand, and she explained to me that she worked as a sister, on a busy surgical ward, in London, for over thirty years.

As her breathing worsened, she squeezed on to my hand tighter. "Am I going to die?" she asked. It is one of the hardest questions I think I was asked up until that point, I had to think very carefully about my answer. "We can talk to the doctor in the visitor's room with you, when your family comes, we can have a discussion about your condition then, but I want you to know I am here for you," I promised.

Katherine smiled at me, but suddenly I was called away to the side room, Clive had called his buzzer and sat frustrated in his chair, "Where are my tablets? I want to go home!" he shouted. "Clive, I have requested your tablets from the pharmacy department, they should be up here shortly," "well if they are not here by 12, I'm gone!" he shot back at me. I felt overwhelmed at times like these, I could not rush the process of promo

I then went back to my own bay to complete my care round, I walked into my bay and in the space of five minutes, Sheila had thrown her bedsheets on the floor, her magazines, clothes, and pens, and lay on the bottom of a disturbed Alana's bed.

"Please can you remove her from my bed, right now please!" warned Alana. I carefully helped Shelia move up in the bed, and helped her return to her bedside, it was then that she required one to one supervision in the bay as she sat in her chair, and a healthcare assistant had to carefully observe her.

I proceeded to have my break, half an hour of fresh air, and going for a walk to the shops, helped to clear my head during a busy shift. When I returned the occupational therapist, Catherine stood with her blue satchel, "right let's go!" she beamed excitedly. We made our way down the hospital stairs to the hospital entrance; I was excited to be visiting a patient's home for the first time.

At the entrance stood the hospital transport driver Clive, he wore a blue boiler suit, he had long curly grey hair and wore bright blue sunglasses. "Where have you been? Your Late!" he scowled. "I'm sorry Clive but I had a phone call to make," Catherine began, "the phone call could have bloody waited I've got a schedule to keep!" Clive shouted. We made our way to Clive's van and put the commode seat and toilet rail in the back of the van, to fit into Alana's toilet at home.

We Stepped into Clive's van, and we were both taken aback at the stale stench in the car, it smelt like rotten vegetables, I quickly rolled the windows down and took in the cold air. It was then that Clive started to turn up the radio full blast. I could see Catherine's face in the mirror contort in anger, "please Clive can you turn it down!" Catherine shouted. I could see Clive's face start to boil red with anger, "what is wrong with you? All you do is moan you are really getting on my nerves!" Clive yelled. "I don't appreciate that tone!" Catherine wined. Sadly, Catherine and Clive's relationship never recovered after the outburst, and they refused to speak to each other.

We pulled up outside of Alana's semidetached house, in a rural part of Yorkshire. At the entrance was Louisa, Alana's estranged daughter who chose to meet us on the visit. As we entered the house we looked on in shock. "Good heavens above," Catherine shouted. As we looked around, we witnessed that the house was full of different colored cats,

We went into the living rooms and found carts crawling all over the sofa and on the mantelpiece, with cat feces all over the rooms. When we went into the kitchen, there were over twenty cats, some crawling on the table, and three little kittens desperately trying to crawl out of the sink, and a few dead cats in the cupboard. We were in shock. "I really didn't things were this bad, Mum has cut us all off you see since Dad died," Louise began crying into her tissue.

We found further evidence that Alana was struggling at home, the food in the fridge had turned to mold, the bathroom was covered in feces, and clothes in her bedroom were piled all over the floor covered in muddy footprints. We were able to fit the commode and bed rail in the bathroom, and Catherine requested for a cleaning service to come and clean the house. When we returned to the hospital it was wonderful to watch Louisa reunite with Alana. Alana had accepted help from Catherine, including the cleaners coming to the house, and to have two care assistants help her each day.

It was then that I realized the Curtains were pulled around Katherine's bed space, my mentor revealed to me that Katherine had passed away whilst I had been on my visit. I worried in case she was alone, I hoped that her family members were with her on in her final moments. I found it so hard losing a patient in my care, it was one of the hardest parts of being a student nurse,

and it reminded me of what I was yet to face with my brother.

The morning after I opened the first envelope, I drove in my brother's red polo

car, to Alnwick, setting out at 6 am in the morning arriving at 8 am. I needed

time to get away from my home, I could not think of the pending funeral in the

upcoming weeks, I needed to escape.

I sat on the rock, overlooking the beautiful bright sea. as the sun glistened, I

had so many memories on the beach, building our first sandcastles together,

playing badminton, and learning to surf.

I wondered if he could see me, if he was watching down on me, if he knew how lonely I was, I felt numb.

I managed to get through the funeral and said my final goodbye, it was so hard seeing Michael's friends and other family members, and I just wanted the day to end. On the night of the funeral, I opened the third envelope that Michael had prepared for me. It was a letter from our estranged Sister Susan.

Susan had cut off all contact with my mother following my parents' divorce, but Michael wanted her to support Mum to visit her In London. It was then I could see the purpose of Michael's letters, the purpose of his 'wishes' was to rebuild our family again once he had passed.

I awoke the next day, and Mum was laying on the couch with Michael's winters coat wrapped around her, Dad was sleeping in the guest room, as Mum asked him to stay for a few days before he had to return to New York. I showed mum the letter Michael and written, she was in shock, and she phoned Susan, and she came to visit that afternoon.

We all sat together in the dining room, with our warm tomato soup, with the log fire burning. We sat and spoke about Michaels adventures as a trainee doctor, and watched home videos of when we went on holiday, including our trip to the Grand Canyon, and watched Michael bungee jumping in Australia on our eighteenth birthday. We sat around the fire talking with blankets wrapped around us, as I turned around to the window ledge, I noticed a single white feather. I felt like it was a message from Michael letting me know he was here.

Chapter 4: The orthopedic ward

During my time as a student nurse, I spent most my time on medical wards, when I found out I was allocated to a busy thirty-five bedded orthopedic ward,

I was happy to finally be introduced to surgical nursing. In the orthopedic department, we had two wards, one was a surgical admission ward, and the second was the post-operative ward.

On my first day, I worked on the admission ward, and I met my mentor Sally. Sally was twenty-four years old and a wild character. She had red hair with blue streaks, and tattoos of the names of all the countries she visited across her arms. "Hello Chris, I'm so excited to meet you, I will be your mentor for the remaining nine weeks, you are my first ever student!" she beamed. "Today you will be admitting patients to theatre, completing a history checklist, I will give you four patients to start with." she cheered.

The admission ward was quite small, with two bays, and was staffed by two nurses. Sally quickly showed me around the ward before assigning me to my jobs. My role was admitting patients, including taking patient observations, helping patients put on their ted compression stockings, and taking patient's clinical history.

I walked into the bay to admit my four patients. The first patient looked extremely familiar, it was my old Irish history teacher of mine Mrs. Oakley, and she was very strict. I always felt nervous looking after patients I knew and living in a small Yorkshire town this was a frequent occurrence.

"Hello Chris, nice to see you, I would never have thought you would become a student nurse, I would have seen you as a hairdresser actually," she giggled. I then presented to her the ted stockings, theatre gown, and hat, "I will help you put on the-"

"No thank you Chris, I am very capable of dressing myself thank you, now there's a buzzer going off, and I think there is a lady in the corner that requires your attention," she added. I felt like I was sixteen again! She clearly found it uncomfortable with me giving her instructions, "Bless him I use to teach him, imagine asking me if I need help," she whispered to the patient next to her, Mrs. Oakley was due to have a knee replacement.

The patient next to Mrs. Oakley was Shelia a forty-five-year-old lady from Birmingham who was admitted having hip surgery. She sat in the chair wearing a grey tracksuit, on her bed, she had a bag filled with chocolates and opened crisp packets. "Hello bab, how are you? "I'm fine I'm Chris I'm here to help prepare you for surgery," I began. I pulled the curtains around and Sheila changed into her gown, and theatre hat.

I then had to help her put on the ted stockings which were thick elasticated socks. I really struggled to put them on, "I'll do it myself Bab," She scowled. Then the consultant walked in Mr. Sharp, "Good morning Sheila I've come to ask you a few questions," He said, before looking with concern at the opened crisp packets. "Have you been eating today?" he asked. "I've had a few crisps and a fry up this morning nothing else," she added. "Mrs. Clarke you will have to postpone your surgery today, you were supposed to remain nil by mouth from 9pm last night," "No one fucking told me, I had to not eat, I had to wait three fucking months for this surgery, there must be something you can do!" she shouted. "Sorry," said Mr sharp walking off.

Sheila then grabbed her items, storming off the ward in anger." As soon as she left Mrs. Oakley stood up and sprayed her air freshener all over Shelia's bed space, "That woman was a foul-mouthed woman who smells worse than a pigsty, good riddance she laughed.

It was then that Sally appeared, skipping into the bay to check on me, as I went to admit Mr Crane, an eighty-nine-year-old man, due to having shoulder surgery. He appeared quite confused, as I completed his observations, he reached his grand round to Sally to pinch her bottom, "I beg your pardon sir," she said. "Sorry lass" he began. I then handed him the gown and net underwear, and ted stockings, and drew the curtains around him for him to get changed.

I waited outside whilst he got changed, and after five minutes I came in and stood in shock. He managed to put the net pans over his head thinking they were a top, and the ted stockings were placed on his arm. I then had to assist him with getting changed, and he suddenly felt dizzy and fell onto the floor. He began to have a panic attack, Sally came in from behind the curtains, and ushered him to the chair, holding his hand and reassuring him that he would be ok.

I then went on to admit my next patient Mrs. Gullah from Iceland. She was unable to speak any English and was admitted for surgery on her knee, which she twisted in a fall. Mrs Gull's daughter Sheena sat next to her, to interpret what she was saying. "Mum said you seem a nice boy," she began. "Mum hasn't been able to walk in thirty years, we are hoping that she will walk following the surgery, she smiled!" it was quite difficult looking after a patient who spoke a different language, and I often hoped the wards would one day employ a translator.

I then proceeded to take the three patients to the theatre one by one for their surgery.

I then spent time at a student induction to complete my manual handling refresher course. I returned to the post-operative ward to care for the patients I admitted.

I had six patients to look after, the first was Mrs. Gullah, the eighty-year-old patient who had wrist surgery, and she lay snoring in the bed.

The second patient was my teacher, Mrs. Oakley, she lay in the bed holding a sick bowl, with the blood pressure cuff attached to her, she was sweating and shivering, common side effects from surgery.

The third patient was Anna, an eighth-year old lady, who had been on the ward for over three months, due to complications in her knee joint surgery. She lay sleeping in her recliner chair, wearing big black orthopedic boots resting on a footrest.

The fourth lady was Trudy, a medical lady admitted as a social admission, as she was struggling to manage at home, she lay in the bed crying, as her elderly husband sat beside her stroking her head.

The fifth patient was Dana a twenty-eight-year-old lady who was waiting to be discharged following total hip surgery.

The final patient I looked after was Mr. Crane he was admitted into the side room, he was too upset and nervous to have his surgery, so they had to postpone it to the next day.

I felt under pressure, Sally had to go to a meeting and left me under the supervision of the senior sister with a checklist of jobs. I had to accurately complete observations every half an hour, monitor urine output, and run back and forth to help the patients go to the toilet.

Mrs. Gullah complained that she was in great pain, her daughter translated to me that she needed to go to the toilet. Suddenly the physiotherapist appeared asking to see Mrs. Gull's level of mobility. She drew the curtains and was able to understand Mrs. Gullah and could communicate to her.

Despite stating she could not mobile for over thirty years she was able to mobilize with ease into the commode chair and was wheeled to the toilet.

Five minutes later ten members of Mrs. Gull's family members entered the ward. The healthcare assistant Tracey started to get angry storming in, "Excuse me there are only two patients allowed to see a patient at a time," she snapped. "Excuse me my mother is critically ill," the daughter shouted. "No, she's not she's only had wrist surgery!" Tracey added, rolling her eyes sarcastically.

It was then that Trudy rang the buzzer, I walked over, and she was sitting up in the bed crying, whilst her frustrated husband sat next to her. "Can you tell him to go he's driving me mad!" she shouted. "Just ignore her son, she's just upset." "No, I'm not Call security, I want him out, he doesn't love me anymore," she cried hysterically. I looked over to the husband, he sat with a carrier bag, full of hospital sandwiches, he had managed to steal at mealtimes. In the handover the nurses claimed that Trudy and her husband had been aggressively fighting at night at home, cultivating in her throwing his cat out of the window of their apartment.

I then went over to Mrs. Oakley my ex-teacher, she looked physically in pain her face was green colored, she kept crying out, even though she was on continuous morphine pain medication. I completed observations and her temperature was over forty degrees, her heart rate was 110 beats per minute and her respirations were high. I contacted the ward doctors who prescribed her fluids, and she started to scream in pain, "I can't breathe someone help me," she yelled. She had to be put on three litters of oxygen to manage her breathing. I sat there and held onto her hand, it felt so strange seeing my ex-teacher, so strong and so in control, now helpless, she held onto my hand and thanked me for helping her.

It was then that the sister on the ward, Sister Criss, called me to the nurse's station where she stood with the physiotherapist and Mrs. Gull's daughter. Mrs. Gull's daughter became very angry and claimed that me and the physiotherapist carried her mother out of the bed, and that she could not possibly walk on her own. "Mrs. Gullah walked around to the chair with a Zimmer frame with minimal assistance," I responded. "You are lying, my mother has been bed-bound for thirty years, she said you both carried her against her will to the chair," she shouted. I could not believe what the daughter was an accusing me of, I stood with the physiotherapist in disbelief.

I then went over to Anna, the patient who had been on the ward for over three months. She had asked me and the healthcare assistant Emily to help her into the bed, we had to use the full hoist. Anna's complications from her knee surgery were so serious, she had been informed that she would never walk again. When we helped her into bed she began to cry, by her bedside was a picture of her husband and daughter, a black and white photo of them making sandcastles. "I've got nothing to live for now I've lost my daughter and husband I want to die!" she shouted.

"Keep positive you will be home soon, you have to stay strong," I smiled trying to be positive. It was then that Emily ushered me over to speak to her, she explained that she had lost her daughter and husband a month ago in a tragic car accident and was adjusting to the prospect of entering a care home.

It was now 6pm, and as I went round to check on my patients, I witnessed that Trudy had the curtains drawn, I peeked in and could see that her husband was devouring one of the several sandwiches he had stolen, and even managed to steal two bowls of sticky toffee pudding.

I went to check on Mrs. Oakley, who was now settled, sitting up in her bed, as the effects of her analgesia had worn off, she was now breathing normally, and her temperature and heart rate had dropped down to the normal ranges.

I felt so busy already on my first day, responding to a patient's critical illness, helping Mrs. Gullah miraculously walk and being involved in a dispute, and successfully admitting patients with little supervision.

Chapter 5: The Community Experience

I remembered how relaxed I was on my community placement, no more 5 am wake up calls, and instead of working long shifts, I would start at 9am, with a warm cup of tea in the district nurse's office, before we set out for the day.

I would always wait with nervous anticipation sitting in my mentor June's beetle, she suffered terribly from road rage and her constant smoking in the car which made me incessantly cough throughout the placement. June had over forty years' experience as a nurse and was the longest service nurse in the district nurse office.

As we drove along the country roads of Yorkshire, June had a banana in one hand a cigarette in her mouth, whilst I held onto the seat as she drove dangerously fast down, swearing throughout.

The first two female patients we went to see did not answer the door, so we made our way to the third house, a seventy-nine-year-old man, who was struggling to cope following his diagnosis of heart failure. We knocked on the door of his ground floor flat. Inside, the house was cluttered with antique ornaments, and awards and medals he won from his days as football captain. In the living room was a green leather sofa with a black and white television situated in the middle of the room.

By the window Geoff's wife lay in her hospital bed, she had advanced stage dementia.

"Well tell me about you how are you coming here with your wife? How are managing self-administering your own medications?" June asked. Geoffrey then brought his blister pack out from his cupboard, which contained all her medications he required in little packets for each day of the week. All the tablets were mixed up in the blister pack, meaning he was not taking the right medications daily.

He then sat on the sofa between me and June, he was over twenty stone and wore a grey vest with black trousers. Geoff's legs and feet were severely swollen, and he had a chronic cough, due to his forty a day smoking habit. Geoff broke down and started crying, "It's so hard managing on my own, my wife use to do the cooking and the household chores, I was the provider, but I'm struggling because she requires help with everything, and I just have no one to help me!" he cried.

"Well we are here to help you, Geoffrey, we can set up a care package so care assistants, can help your wife, and to make sure you take the right medication, you are not alone," Jean reassured him, placing her hand gently onto his. "It's so lonely and isolating I have no one to talk to here, I feel depressed," he managed. "We can offer you a befriender, someone who volunteers to help you with your shopping each day, and can come around to talk to you, how does that sound? June asked.

"Fantastic" Geoffrey applied, crying into Junes Shoulder. It was then I saw the true essence of being a nurse, making a difference to a person's life through providing support and going the extra mile.

It was then that we proceeded to carry on with her journey, June drove along the country road, singing 'Born in the USA,' before pulling up to a little semidetached house next to the town center. "Right Chris we can just make a little pit stop to John's house, I promised to see him," she smiled. John had been part of June's previous client base for over twenty years, but June wanted to visit him to offer him a haircut! She brought in her bag of supplies, her scissors, and hair creams and proceeded to cut John's hair in his kitchen, whilst I looked on in awe. We had slightly deviated from our duties that morning!

The next patient we went to visit was Deidre, an eighty-three-year-old lady, she had recently been diagnosed with Parkinson's disease, we entered her flat, which was on the top floor of a ten-story block of flats. When we entered the small flat, Deidre lay on the living room floor with her head against the sofa. Deirdre had a facial droop, her speech was slurred and incomprehensible, and she was unable to move her limbs. We positioned Deidre to keep her comfortable before calling the ambulance team.

Deidre had suffered from a severe stroke and was taken instantly to the A and E department. The ambulance team explained that we got to Deidre just in time, if she had been left on the floor any longer, she may not have survived her stroke.

It was a valuable experience as a student nurse, looking after patients in the community. Although without the other members of staff, the nurses, care assistants, and doctors, you really felt as if you were on your own, especially in emergencies, and had a lack of equipment to deal efficiently with emergency situations.

At 2 pm that afternoon we arrived at Ashbourne clinic. Every Thursday, June would work in the clinic as a practice nurse, assisting patients with injections, leg dressings, and offered health promotion. I sat nervously in the clinic, whilst a concerned June looked at me, "Don't be so fucking nervous, you always look scared out of your wits, patients are not going to bite you." she warned. It was in that clinic that we saw a range of patients, ranging from a man who required compression leg bandaging, to a girl who came in to discuss her pregnancy diagnosis and a man who came for advice, over managing his type one diabetes condition. Many of the patients had known June for a long time, but June could only help them with one health issue, as many patients came in with multiple health problems.

I enjoyed my time in the community, I had spent two placements in a hospital setting, and working with the district nurses felt like a welcome break, from the stress-free environment of the ward. It was during the community placement that my brothers condition rapidly declined, I would arrive home at 4 pm, and he would be asleep with the television still on. Sometimes at night, his condition would deteriorate, and we often spent many nights in the A and E department, to help Michael cope with the effects of his treatment.

It felt so great having Susan back in our lives after we spent the evening talking around the fire, I woke up the next day from a phone call from my mentor on the medical ward. She had invited me to come back to the ward to finish my final placement and offered her condolences on my brothers passing. I was still unsure what to do, I was still waiting for a phone call regarding my audition, but I knew I had to keep busy, and could not spend all my time grieving.

That morning Dad had a surprise for us all, he had spent all night in the garage pumping up the tires of our old old mountain bikes. When I was younger, we would often all go on bike rides, and have a picnic in Everfield Forest in Yorkshire.

Dad had requested that we go on a final bike ride before he headed off to Birmingham airport for his flight home. It took much persuasion, but we managed to encourage mum out of the house, it had been over two weeks since she left the house. We were soon rushing through the town on our mountain bikes, the hot winters sun glistened as we traveled through the streets. It was the perfect day, we had a picnic on a hill in Everson Forest, Mum and Susan lay out the picnic blanket, soaking up the hot sun, and reminiscing about better times. I then want up to Everson Lake with Dad and we went fishing, it was the perfect afternoon. It felt like our family was being reconnected again, it made it even more distressing that Dad was leaving that day.

At 6 pm we all waved goodbye, as Dad disappeared in the taxi, as we watched him go, I watched Mum as she quickly went into the dining room to book a taxi, "I have to tell your father something I can't let him go!" she warned, she quickly grabbed her winters coat, and called a taxi.

I went upstairs to open the final envelope from Michael, the final wish, and nothing could prepare me for what I was about to find.

Chapter 6: Pathways

After the community placement, I was sent by the university to my pathway placement, it was three weeks in an ophthalmology eye clinic followed by two weeks in a diabetes treatment clinic.

I remember how busy the eye clinic was, as soon as I entered, the waiting area was full of waiting patients, there were over ten clinic rooms in the eye clinic, which included nurse consultation rooms and doctors' rooms. It was then that I met my supervisor Kashwere who trained as a nurse in Canada, she was six foot tall with wild curly ginger hair. "Hello I am Kashwere welcome to the

Yorkshire community eye clinic," She shouted. I never understood why she spoke with such a loud tone.

I shadowed Kashwere in the morning in the clinic. I watched as she completed visual field tests on the patients, checking for any changes in their vision. I remember one patient at 89, who came in at only four foot five, when Ashwere attempted to administrate the eye drops she kept blinking repeatedly, and let out a scream, when the eye drops managed to reach her eyes. Several patients had shown how they found it difficult to administer eye drops at home, with one lady who suffered with Glaucoma and self-administered the eye drops in front of Ash Were claiming that she 'gives them a good go,' instead poring the eye drop all over her forehead.

Ashwere explained that she grew up in Africa, and came to England at sixteen to start a better life for her. She worked as an auxiliary nurse before completing her training ten years later. Ashwere seemed to ask me so many questions, 'Why do you want to be a nurse?' 'Tell me everything you know about the anatomy of the eye?' When I went to the staffroom and made myself a cup of tea, I could hear two nurses in the background, "I can't believe how rude Ashwere was this morning, barging into my clinic room asking for help," moaned the nurse. "Remember we have to keep a written record of her behavior," continued the other nurse.

It was then that I observed a patient having their weekly Lucentis injections, and I had to practice the non-touch technique putting on the gloves, Ashwere put them on with ease after twenty years of practice. With all eyes on me I attempted to put the gloves on but instead snapped and broke the gloves in my nervousness, by the third attempt I finally was able to put the gloves on.

On my pathway in the eye clinic, I worked with patients who had a range of eye problems such as glaucoma, cataracts, and severe dry eyes. Many Patients with severe eyesight loss would walk in with walking sticks and frames, and it made me realize how truly grateful I was for having good eyesight. It felt like the longest two weeks being in the eye clinic, in my time there I completed only one visual field test and administered eye drops to one other patient. I soon discovered I am a person who likes to be actively involved in the workplace and observing can become tedious after fourteen days.

My time at the diabetes clinic was more productive. I was working with Shelley a forty-year-old nurse, with over eighteen years of nursing experience. in the clinic, we met with patients who were suffering from type one and type 2 diabetes. It was a busy clinic, in which we had to give treatment plans and health advice to patients diagnosed with diabetes.

I remember one patient John aged thirty-two, who had been diagnosed with type 2 diabetes, he admitted his daily diet included a fry up in the morning, three sandwiches for lunch, a curry or fish and chips for dinner, and over ten mars bars, and multiple fizzy drinks during the day. John admitted that his poor diet was due to depression, and that food helped to fill the void following his divorce. The hba1c test that Shelley demonstrated to me showed the level of blood sugar in his body over a three-month period, which was very high. Shelley asked if he could help to monitor his diet, by reducing the amount of carbohydrates, and having an equal amount of proteins and fiber in his diet and looked at alternative sugar alternatives.

John Admitted that due to being unemployed and his lack of social interaction, he was going to find it about having very hard to change his diet as food brought him comfort. It was then that Shelley offered him a leaflet to join a local community cricket club, as cricket was one of John's strong interests. Shelley also spoke to John about commencing on insulin. When he left Shelley admitted that she found it very difficult giving patients a new diagnosis of diabetes, and often worried of the effects on their health if they did not follow her recommendations.

I remember a twenty-one-year-old patient, Thomas, that Shelley had looked after for over ten years, he had suffered with type one diabetes. He was a famous Olympic runner, but over the years he had been struggling to manage this condition. "It used to be so hard to remember to take my insulin, due to being on the running track from 6 am each morning, and my running schedule seemed to overtake my life. Since I have had my insulin pump my life has changed forever," he smiled. It was then that Tom revealed the insulin pump which delivers continuous insulin throughout the day. "It really has changed my life I no longer need to worry about taking my medication, it truly has allowed me to live an independent life," he added.

As a student I had learned so much in the diabetes clinic, and how the condition affected patients over a long-term period. Some of the elderly patients suffered from eye conditions such as macular degeneration, whilst others were treated for foot ulcers, and some patients had secondary conditions, that coexisted with their diabetes such as heart failure.

I had learned so much from Shelley who imparted her knowledge onto me, and let me take blood sugars and become involved in the clinics. Sometimes on the ward and in the eye clinic, I felt like there were some nurses who seen a student as a 'chore' and tended to use me as an extra pair of hands and were too busy to mentor me due to their management responsibilities. In order to get the best out of your placement as a student nurse, your mentor must be receptive to helping you, as you cannot learn alone.

I walked nervously into my room and opened the final envelope, it had a pair

of keys inside, with my Grandparents address scrawled on a note. 'Here is the

key to something special' read the note. I wondered what it meant, could it be that Michael had bought our old Grandparents' house and renovated it? I was determined and eager to discover the meaning.

That evening, Mum returned with Dad to the house, I sat on the couch in confusion with Susan. "I went to the airport to explain to your Father that I want him around a little longer, we are going to try and work things out," she smiled, holding onto Dad's hand. I sat in shock at mum's submission. "What about your home in New York, your job?" Susan asked. "All of that does not matter, Michael's passing made me realize how important family is, and I want to be happy again" he added.

That evening I had to explain to Mum, Dad, and Susan that Michael had left envelopes with wishes in to help me through this time. I presented the keys and my grandparents address to my parents. "We should all go and see what surprised he has instore for us," Dad began. "I thought you sold their cottage, could he have really bought the cottage?" I asked. "Well, he worked since he was sixteen, and he had a lot of money saved, there must be a reason," Mum added.

We all agreed that night that we would visit the cottage on the weekend, at the time I believed that this was Michael's final wish, but he was not finished with communicating with us yet.

Chapter 7: The Demon Mentor

I remember when I first discovered I was going to be working in a theatre department. I had spent six months in a ward at this point and was unprepared for the challenges I would face. The theatre placement was about to be the most difficult placement I ever endured, and the negative effects that occurred, stay with me to this day.

I was completing the placement with another student nurse called Laura. Our mentor was Helen, a theatre nurse who despised student nurses, and saw them as insects she wanted to squash. She was six-foot-tall, with long curly blond hair, green demon eyes and walked like a dictator.

I remember when we were introduced to her the theatre staff who were completing their handover, and she took us into a small office. "Hello, I am Helen I will be your mentor, here is a reading list, today I will orientate you into the theatre and the next shift we can hit the ground running." she smiled. That day we observed a variety of surgeries including plastic surgery and orthopedic surgery.

On my second shift, I worked in close proximity with my mentor and that is when the nightmare began. We worked in the recovery department, it was a cold room with white walls and three beds ready in the stations to take to theatre. I remember sitting on the stool and Helen began to fire questions at me 'name all the bones in the body' 'explain the function of the endocrine system,' I didn't have a chance to revise on all of the questions and she shot an angry look at me, "You have a lot of work to do, I will test tomorrow," she scowled.

It was then that we had to collect our patient from theatre, it was an orthopedic patient who had just had knee surgery. Helen removed the breathing tube and performed suctioning on the patient. I then had to record the patient observations every five minutes. She came to look at my observations standing over me, "Hurry up you have to be quicker than that," she sneered. Then it was time to move the patient in the bed to reposition them, "Have you mobilized an orthopedic patient before?" she asked "yes" I responded. She then proceeded to grab my hands forcefully putting them onto the patient angrily. I felt like I was assaulted, I knew that I was working with a very dangerous character.

The nurses from the theatre then brought out a second patient who had a gastric band insertion, "Go and take the observations now, and this time I'm timing you," she whined. I went over to the next patient to take the patient observations. Helen asked me to explain the ABC assessment technique, something I had revised, which she responded I needed to improve my technique.

As time continued the placement, I felt like I was a prisoner, rather than a student nurse. I was in the presence of a very troubled woman, who thrived on degrading me, belittling me, and someone who loved to destroy a student's confidence. By the end of the placement my mentor's bullying was so extreme that I would visibly shake on the ward, and to no surprise, to me I failed my placement even in areas I had passed before.

If I had spoken up at the start of the placement, the individual would never have been able to carry out her wicked actions. Ever since I completed the placement, I always encouraged student nurses to speak up if they feel bullied, as the way the mentor treated me has stayed with me ever since it is important to always have the courage to speak up. I since discovered that my mentor bullied an experienced sister in another ward, it is still to this day one of the worst experiences of my life to suffer and endure.

Chapter 8: Work Experience

I remembered my time back in the summer of 2013, completing bank work in different wards. I felt it was great experience working on different wards, but often challenging, whilst working without the safety net of a mentor. My first bank shift was on Aspen ward, a medical ward in south Yorkshire. As soon as I entered the handover the sister was panicking, as one nurse and healthcare assistants had called in sick, leaving only four members of staff on the ward.

There were twenty-one patients on the ward, and I was asked to supervise a bay of four patients who required constant supervision, due to the high risk of them falling. The patients included Arthur an eighty-two-year-old, aggressive man, with advanced dementia. He had been on the ward for over three months, as the ward staff struggled to find a nursing placement for him. The second gentlemen were Ashley an eighty-nine-year-old man with recent confusion, he lay peacefully in the bed. The man opposite him was a young man who was under investigation after mysterious red blotches appeared over his body, and he was sent to the ward for investigation. The man next to him was Jim a 90-year-old man, who was an ex-soldier, who lost both legs in the Second World War, and suffered from advanced Parkinson's disease.

I felt more relaxed during my bank work and felt less pressure, my job was to supervise the patients, provide personal care, and assist them to mobilize.

I began by looking through the patient's folders, to check their mobility. All of a sudden, an unsteady Arthur stood up in his chair, I quickly ran over to him providing him with the Zimmer frame, "Go away you bastard I don't need a frame, I can walk to the toilet myself," he argued, kicking the frame out of sight, I then had to hold his hand as he struggled to walk to the toilet. I had to call the nurse to supervise my patients in the bay.

As I walked into the toilet with the patient, I offered to stand by the curtain to help if he needed, but he refused my offer, carefully pushing me out of the toilet before locking it. After five minutes of persistent knocking I opened the door and looked on in horror.

An explosion of diarrhea occurred, smeared all over the toilet, the sink, and even on the walls, the patient's brown handprint was all over the wall and brown footprints appeared all over the floor. I didn't know whether to laugh or cry, I called the other healthcare assistant who took the patient to the shower room for a wash, then had I had to proceed with a mop to clean up the disastrous mess, whilst trying hard not to cry. "Next time we will bring a commode to the toilet, he shouldn't have gone to the toilet," muttered the nurse. Arthur walked to the bed and fell asleep within minutes.

Suddenly Ashley woke up next to him, "what is your name? Where do you come from?" he asked. "I work here, I'm here to help you," I began. I investigated the bed and realized he had poured the water onto his sheets, they were soaked. Along with the other nurse we tried to help him to get comfortable, by changing him into his pajamas, he resisted to turn in the bed, he began to hit out at us, and shouted, "Help they are killing me!" We waited until he calmed down, and he began to throw his book, his water jug, and coins onto the bay floor in frustration.

The young patient Jason looked on helplessly, and with frustration, as he desperately tried to sleep that night. Jim had been awake for over two days. I sat at the desk, filing in the care round and repositioning charts. I had been on the ward for three hours and had no time to even have a drink of water. I had to constantly keep a close watch on the patients at all times. As I completed my notes, I looked on in shock as Jim the ex-war hero had managed to get out

of bed and proceeded to crawl across the floor, I looked at the desperation on

his face, "Jim let me help you back to your bed it's not safe," "I'll give you safe

just hop it, go on clear off!" he barked angrily. The nurses watched as he made

his way to the toilet with his face boiling red with determination.

As soon as he returned I found it hard keeping an eye on all of the three

patients, Arthur repeatedly tried to get out of bed and walk unaided to the

toilet, I had to consistently assure Ashley that he was in the hospital, and to

help place his legs in the bed, as he consistently tried to get out of bed, whilst

Jim sang repeatedly in the bed, disturbing the other patients. It is a tough

challenge to watch three patients throughout a twelve-hour shift, I felt a lot of

pressure, but managed to make it through.

My next shift was at the Yorkshire sleep clinic, I completed an eight-hour shift

from 10pm to 6 am in the morning. The sleep clinic was a booked in service, in

which patients were sent to following a referral by the doctor. The office

contained a big CCTV screen, which allowed healthcare workers to observe the patients and check their vital signs. We had two patients booked into the sleep clinic both suffering from narcolepsy. I attached them to the leads which helped to monitor their sleeping pattern. As I sat in the office another healthcare assistant entered the room, "excuse me who are you what are you doing" "I'm Chris I was booked here," I began. "There is only meant to be one person on here!" she groaned. After her initial frustration, Hayley managed to sit down. I tried desperately to stay awake, I felt so tired just sitting down watching the screen. A few hours later one of the patients jumped up and pressed the buzzer, and we both fought to help assist him to the toilet. The sleep clinic was a very different environment in comparison to the ward. I realized once I was working there, that working on the ward environment was for me, I enjoyed hands-on nursing and working as part of a busy team.

Saturday came around quickly, and we all packed our belonging to travel to Alnwick to discover Michael's surprise. Keeping busy as a family helped us in our grief, going on the bike ride, and now taking a family trip helped us all, it was so easy to want to stay in bed and hide under the covers, but we faced it as a family.

I packed my scrapbook that Michael made me, and my diary, and a few casual outfits. We went in Dad's green jeep, and traveled the two-hour journey to Alnwick, no one spoke in the car, and Susan fell asleep next to me, whilst mum played Sudoku on her phone. I reached for my phone in my satchel, and realized I had two phone calls, one from the theatre in New York, and one phone call from my previous mentor on the cardiology ward.

My heart pounded with fear, and then seconds later the phone battery died. I realized that now was not the time to discover the fate of my future, I had to see what Michael had planned for us. An hour later we arrived at our Grandparents cottage, on the hill next to fox ton beach. The cottage was painted blue, with a red door. As we apprehensively made our way to the cottage, there was a plague with all our initials attached to it. We entered the cottage and looked on in amazement. The living room had a king size black leather couch, a fifty-inch plasma screen was attached to the wall. A family photo taken over ten years ago of our family having a picnic on Foxton beach with all of us having a barbeque on the beach hung above the fireplace. The conservatory had a large ten-meter hot tub, the kitchen had a grand Victorian table, and upstairs the four guest bedrooms were renovated, each one had a king size bed and a television in each room.

Mum stood in the hallway in shock, "How did he do this? He couldn't have renovated the cottage on his own," Mum gasped. "I helped," Susan admitted. "I helped cover the costs, he wanted to create a family holiday home, and he wanted you all to be happy here." Susan cheered.

Mum stood and smiled; it was the first time I saw her smile since Michael passed.

I had charged my phone and walked nervously to fox ton beach, it was a windy afternoon, the sand blew across my face, and the waves crashed against the sea. I sat trembling as I lay in the sand, I reached into my pocket and listened to the answer phone message, it was from John the judge in the New York theatre company. My hand trembled as he began to speak, 'I'm sorry to tell you your audition for the role of the scarecrow was unsuccessful.' That was it.

After making the journey to New York and following my acting dream, and following my brothers wish, my fate was sealed by a single sentence.

I did not have the heart to tell my family what happened, I wanted everyone to enjoy their break. I sat down with my family and we enjoyed our roast dinner. I had to keep strong despite the bad news.

Chapter 9: The final placement

Following on from the week of being at the cottage, I had finally come to terms with failing the audition of my dreams, I now had to keep positive and look forward. I rang my Mentor Kate from my final placement. and she agreed that I could come back and finish my final four weeks of the placement.

I started back on my placement on Monday 1st April, I woke up at 5am, and quickly prepared my satchel with my lunch, and water bottle, and my notebook. I put my white student nurse uniform on, and I was ready to go. I walked nervously to the hospital that morning and crept with great trepidation onto the ward.

As soon as I entered, I could hear the beeping of the observation machines, and cardiac monitors, the loud ringing of the patient buzzers, and the night staff rushing around making sure they completed their final tasks. The ward was the same, but I felt like a different person, gone was the confident enthusiastic person I once was, I was now filled with fear.

I entered the staffroom at 7am, my mentor Katie was in them along with Susan a newly qualified nurse, Elizabeth a senior nurse, Sister Rebecca, and the healthcare assistants Keeley and Lauren.

After we completed the handover my mentor Kate grabbed me by the hand. "I know you have had such a difficult time, but I have every faith in you that you will be a nurse, that's why I want you to start managing the bay on your own from today, I will act as your healthcare assistant," She smiled. It was my mentor's positivity that kept me going, it made me feel like I could achieve anything.

I walked towards my bay; I was looking after six patients. The first patient was Marjorie an 89-year-old woman who was suffering from respiratory failure and was in the final stages of her condition. The second lady was Dawn a 90-year-old lady with advanced dementia who was sent to hospital, as the nursing home struggled with her behaviour, she was awaiting a new placement. The third patient was Katie, a twenty-four-year-old lady admitted with Sepsis who was awaiting discharge after making a full recovery. The fourth patient was Agatha a seventy-year-old lady admitted with confusion.

Then I also had to take care of the two male patients in the side room. The first patient was Matthew a forty-four-year-old man admitted following a collapse from an undiagnosed heart murmur. The man in the second side room was Augustus, a seventy-five-year-old man admitted with dementia and was obsessed with westerns.

I completed my medication round with Kate, carefully recalling the effects and uses of each medication, as part of my assessment. Medication rounds can always be difficult, when patients refuse tablets, for example Dawn threw the tablets on the floor claiming they were poison, whilst Augustus in the side room, said he will take his tablets only if I let me leave the ward.

We proceeded to wash the patients in the bay. Margery the palliative patient required full assistance to turn in the bed and needed help with washing all areas. I remember her smiling face as she looked up at me, "I'm not going to die, am I?" she questioned. "You just stay strong, I am here to look after you, keep positive," I added, whilst holding her hand.

We then proceeded to wash Dawn who consented to our help, until suddenly, she slapped Kate on the side of her face, "bloody bitches what you are doing to me?"

"I'm trying to help you with a wash Dawn," "No you're not you're after my money! Where's my purse you are thieving bitch!" she scowled. Then Dawn proceeded to grab Kate by the hand, and she dug her sharp fingernails into her. Kate let out a scream and required four healthcare workers to help remove Dawn's grip.

As we finished the wash Katie, the young patient sat in her chair, dressed in her warm winters coat with her suitcase packed, sitting on her bed was a confused Agatha in her red nightdress. "So, when will my tablets be ready, how long will it take? She asked.

 "We have notified pharmacy it shouldn't be too long of a wait," I replied.

"Wait! That's all I've heard since yesterday, if the tablets are not here by twelve, I'm self-discharging," Katie scowled. "Oh, can I self-discharge too," added an excited Agatha.

As I made my way to the nurse station with Kate, we discussed how difficult the shift was at present, with the aggression at the hands of the patients, and the persistent pleads to be discharged. The buzzer went off in the side room, it was Matthew the young patient, he was lying in his bed in his blue tracksuit, clutching a packet of cigarettes in his hands. "Please Chris can I go out for a cigarette please, can you help me," he pleaded. "I'm a little busy at the minute Matthew, maybe when your family arrive, they can take you down to the smoking shelter," I added. He huffed and puffed at my response, but I could not abandon my bay to take a patient outside for a cigarette, and he was already on nicotine patches to help with his condition, and he was warned of the damage further smoking would cause to his condition.

I then went into Augustus room to help complete a leg dressing of the ulcer on his leg. Augustus was a big fan of western films, and on his table, he had several horse figures lined up, and cowboys all in a line on the table. I proceeded to pick up one of the action figures , and Augustus quickly snatched it from my hand, "God bless us and save us, don't take that away from me, they are very precious, I've had these action figures for over 100 years he," he cried.

Augustus consented to me helping him complete his leg dressing, and then his wife arrived Karen, she was an 89-year-old frail lady, walked in with two walking sticks. "Oh no what do you want?" he shouted. It was then that Karen began to cry, as she grabbed me by the shoulders, "he just hates me, every time I come to see him, he's aggressive," she managed, as tears streamed down her eyes. "Augustus do you want to sit with your wife for a while and have a cup of tea?" I offered. Augustus then proceeded to get up from his armchair and walked out of the room, before whispering in my ear, "tell her to sit in the chair, and then you can show me the way out," he began, he then walked over to Karen and held her by the hands. Karen wiped her tears and began to smile, "Oh Augustus I have missed you at home, how have you been?" she looked up at him, full of hope.

"Look darling I don't have a clue that you are, but if you want to sit on the chair and leave me alone, I'd be grateful" he shouted. My mentor Kate took a flustered Augustus by the hand to the nurse's station. I sat with Karen in the side room. I invited her to a case conference, which would take place the next day, in which she could talk about her husband's condition with the doctors, and discuss a nursing home placement, and possible counselling for her deteriorating mental health.

When working with patients with dementia in the hospital it is important to get to know the patient, as each patient's dementia is different to the next patient. Some patients would be aggressive, whilst others would sleep all day, and say very little. It can be very difficult to meet the needs of patients with dementia when their behaviour is unpredictable, and as a student nurse you soon realise the devastating pressures looking after a person with dementia can cause on a family unit.

During the shift the patients in the other bays had made a complaint about how many of their items seemed to go missing, books, glasses, wallets, even items of clothes had disappeared from patient cupboards.

However, the culprit was about to be revealed.

As I went into my bay, I saw Agatha sitting on her chair dressed in a green suit with yellow high heels. Next to her was a suitcase full to the brim. "Right here you are, now then help me carry by bag to the station," she began passing me her suitcase which was now very heavy. "I can't take you home Agatha you need to stay here until you get better," I warned. "Anymore backchat from you and I will call your superior, I'm going home and that is final ok?" she warned.

It was then that Agatha's suitcase burst open, we then witnessed that her suitcase was filled with a range of items she had taken from the other patients, including men's shoes, glasses, bras, magazines and even one of the patient's wedding rings. Kate came into the bay and helped me to put the stolen items into a black bag, much to the anger of Agatha, "what the heck are you doing with all my stuff they are mine," she shouted. "They are not yours Agatha, they belong to the other patients." Kate murmured. Agatha sat in her chair clearly distressed from what she had witnessed, and she began to cry hysterically.

An hour later Agatha, was visited by a mental health nurse who undertook a mental health assessment and she failed each question. She believed the year was 1980, she though Margaret thatcher was the current prime minister, she was unable to recall information, and complete simple calculations. It was suspected that she had the early onset condition of Dementia but was sent for a CT scan to further prove this.

I then had to complete the care round, which included taking the blood pressure heart rate and temperature of all the patients, and repositioning and cleaning patients who required assistance.

I went into the side room to take Matthew's observation he had a mew score of 5. A MEWS score is the total score of all the observation readings. As Matthews's score was 5, I had to now alert the critical care outreach team, who would come to review his condition, his heart rate was over 105 beat per minutes, and his respiration rate was over 24, much over the suspected

reading. I quickly rang the critical outreach team, and explained that Matthew

was tachycardic, and that he was struggling to breathe, and that he appeared

confused.

After the phone call Margery pressed the buzzer, she was laying in her bed

covered in a sea of blankets. Tears were streaming down her face, as reached

out her hands to grab mine, "Oh Chris please don't let me die, you'll help me

won't you, my family couldn't cope without me," she warned. It was then that

she squeezed my hand tightly, "I'm so afraid," she whispered. I looked over

towards her as tears streamed from her face, I could see that she was in pain,

but she was fighting with all her might not to closer her eyes. She worried if

she went to sleep, she would not wake up.

Then her twin sisters Felicia and Nuala entered the war in their matching blue

denim jackets. Marjorie felt a sense of comfort seeing her family members and

it seemed to ease her worries.

I then made myself a desk in the middle of the bay to complete my notes as Kate went for her break. It was now 3pm, It was hard to concentrate, the phone on the nurse's desk seemed to ring constantly, I felt myself ease dropping into family conversations, and I was often pestered with the question 'Are You free'? It was so difficult to concentrate on the hospital ward. As I sat in the middle of the bay, I thought about how different my life would have been if I would have been given the part of the scarecrow in the wizard of oz. I could have got a flat in New York, performed to thousands of patrons each night, and go ice skating every evening.

I had nearly completed my notes, before I could hear the emergency buzzer ring. It was from side room one Matthews's room. I rushed over and witnessed Matthew laying on the floor unconscious on the bed. The healthcare assistant stood over him in shock, "I just came in and he was laying on the floor. I knelt and discovered he was not breathing, and I could not feel a pulse. I started to complete compressions.

Soon a crowd of doctors, nurses and physiotherapists joined me, each taking it in turn to complete the emergency compressions. I stood watching on in guilt, wondering if I had done enough, believing that he may have felt anxiety not being able to have the cigarette he desired. The doctors used the defibrillator on Matthew, but despite their best efforts he died at 3pm. Matthew had died of a heart attack. After confirmation of Michael's death, we helped him onto the bed. Then I found Kate's hand on my shoulder, "you did all you can Chris, you tried your best and I am proud of you," she beamed.

I then went on my half an hour lunch break and quickly devoured my cheese sandwich, and quenched my thirst, with my large hot chocolate with cream. Amongst all the chaos and drama on the ward that day, I seemed to not have had the time, to focus on my own health and to stop and have a drink.

As I returned to the ward, the staff was commending me on my efforts, in taking the command in an emergency, to help the staff.

Katie had finally been discharged after waiting 'forever' for her tablets! Marjorie lay sleeping in her bed, whilst her sisters sat beside her, "She must be exhausted, she keeps dozing in and out of her sleep, it looks like you have a fighter on your hand," Nuala cheered.

I walked over to Agatha who lay on the top of her bed clutching onto her teddy bear, "I want to go home, I want to see my family," she cried. "You just concentrate on having a rest now, you have had a difficult day," I began.

It was then that Kate revealed that she had heard back a negative response from summer nursing home, regarding the placement for Dawn. Dawn's family had hoped that she would reside in the care home, but after visiting the ward, the care team decided that her behaviour was too aggressive, and that she was a risk to the other patients. The negative effect of this, could mean that the patient could stay unnecessarily in the hospital, when medically her condition was stable.

It was now 6pm, and was a quiet time on the ward, the patients were settled and made comfortable in the bed, and I was ready to handover to the night staff. "How do you think you have done today?" Kate asked. "I tried my best," I replied. "Well the ward Manager Maureen wants to see you," she explained.

I instantly thought the worse, believing I had done something wrong. I walked nervously to Maureen's office. The ward manager had over forty years' experience in the NHS and trained in America to complete her nurse training.

"Hello Chris, take a seat I've been looking forward to speaking to you," she smiled. Maureen sat smiling she wore her blue matrons' uniform with the red belt across her chest, she had tanned skin and blonde curly hair was wrapped neatly into a bun. "I just want to say welcome back, and I want to tell you that there is a vacancy for a nurse on our ward in September, and I would love you to be a part of our team."

"That would be wonderful," I beamed, accepting the offer of employment.

I enjoyed being back on the ward and keeping busy, instead of focusing on my grief. The next few weeks were tough, but I managed to get through. I had to pass all my competencies, to prove I met the standards of being a nurse. Susan must travel back to Devon as she was in a senior position as an architect. Mum and Dad were closer than ever, Dad had resigned from his job as a vet in New York and gained a position at a new practice in Yorkshire.

Although we were all still in our deep stages of grief, we were all trying best to move forward in our lives.

A week before the final week of placement I received a phone call from the theatre company of which I auditioned for the role of the scarecrow. "Hello, is that Chris button," said the muffled voice on the end of the phone. "Yes," I panicked, scared and unsure as to what they wanted.

"This is John from Jones theatre company; I'm ringing regarding your audition for the role of scarecrow." said the muffled voice. "I realize I didn't get that part." I murmured. "Well there's been a change of plan, Jason who gained the role of scarecrow has pulled out of the position. We have decided not to audition again for the role, as you really stood out, we want to give you the role," he replied.

"I'll take it!" I beamed.

I was so happy, I always knew it was my destiny to be an actor, and it was Michael's wish for me to follow my dreams, but I had a commitment to finish my nursing course first.

Chapter 10: Transition to a nurse

I was so nervous on Monday, the final day of my placement. It was assessment day, the day I would find out if I meet the requirements to register as nurse. As I walked onto the ward, I realised all the patients I had previously looked after on Friday had now been discharged, so I had to now prove myself with a new bay of patients.

After handover I walked into the bay of six acutely ill male patients.

The first patient was Steven a forty-three-year-old man admitted for alcohol detox, secondary to a stroke. He was bed pound at present and was refusing to comply with physiotherapy treatment.

The next patient was Eden an eight-year-old man with stage three pancreatic cancer, who received all his medication through a syringe driver. The third patient was Donald a seventy-nine-year-old man, who was admitted following a fall at home, and was struggling to cope following the death of his wife.

The fourth patient was Peter a fifty-year-old man admitted following collapsing at a local McDonald's, which was related to the stress from his job as a deputy head teacher. The fifth man Donald aged sixty was waiting for his discharge, after self-admitting himself into the emergency department, after being unable to control his diabetes condition.

The sixth patient was Mal an eight five-year-old man, admitted following becoming increasingly aggressive to the patients in the nursing home.

I had highlighted my handover sheet of the key parts of the patients past medical history, and in my notebook, I compiled a list of the key tasks to be completed on the shift, including, discharges, referral to the dementia team, leg dressings, and delegation for the health care assistants, to assist me with the basic care in my bay. Today was my final day to prove myself as a student nurse, whilst Kate watched from the side-lines.

I had to firstly delegate tasks to the healthcare assistant in my bay Michelle. I found it difficult to delegate and to be in charge as a student nurse, I was quite shy and reserved. I delegated Michelle to give wash bowls to the patients who were able to care for themselves, whilst I worked alongside Michelle to help wash Steven and Donald, who required full assistance with care.

First, we assisted Michael with his wash he struggled to turn in the bed and required full assistance to wash as he refused to comply with the physiotherapists to help with his mobility. It was believed Steve suffered stroke dew to his bad diet and drug use.

The doctors believed that the stroke had such a strong effect on his brain that he may not be able to regain his cognition or speech again. After we assisted him with the wash, I asked him if he wanted us to help him mobilize on the ward. "I don't need any help any help, go away!" he shouted. "Please Steven I want to help you," I pleaded. "Fuck off" he shouted. It was times like this, that I didn't blame the patient for their aggressive actions, he had suffered a major stroke. I referred Steven to the counselling team to help deal with the underlying depression he exhibited.

I then proceeded to wash Malachy he was suffering from dementia, he had signs all over the walls next to his bed such as 'you are at the hospital' 'your son will see you at 3pm' 'press your buzzer if you need the toilet.

We then proceeded to wash him, "hello I am Chris, and this is Michelle we are going to help with your wash this morning," "I need a shave," he replied. We proceeded to pass Malachy the flannels, and he managed to complete his wash and dressing task independently. "I need a shave," he repeated constantly. Although at times as a student you do have to indeed help patients with a shave. I was often wary of using a razor on the skin of elderly gentlemen. I worried in case I would cut into their skin accidently.

It was then that the sister Bridget came towards me. Sister Bridget was a revolutionary sister, a 'true nurse.' At the start of every shift she would greet every patient and make sure they were comfortable, then for the staff huddle she would bring out a tray of tea and toast.

She worked so hard to improve the wellbeing of the staff; however, her only downfall was supporting volunteers on the ward. "Hi Chris, I hope you don't mind Shantell is a six-form student interested in completing her nursing can she shadow you?" she asked. Why are you asking me this! Of all days to ask me, I thought.

"Ok" I agreed. Shantell looked up at me, she had wild red hair, and her face was pale. She seemed so nervous and frightened and did not ask questions or engage with the patients.

I completed the discharge paperwork for Peter the patient who came onto the word following a collapse, I was pleased to report to him that his CT scan results came back normal, and that he was free to go. He had already packed his belongings into his satchel, and he almost ran past me to escape the ward!

Suddenly I heard a loud thud in the bathroom, I quickly ran in with Michelle, the patient Donald had fallen onto his back on the toilet, after tripping on his stick. I quickly took his blood pressure, and along with Michelle we used a hoist to help mobilise him from the bathroom floor to the armchair.

It is always such a traumatic event when a patient fall, it was one of the leading causes for entry into hospitals for elderly people over 65. Once Donald was placed into the chair, I asked Michelle to sit beside him and monitor him in the bay, to help prevent a further fall, I also referred him to the therapy cream to help improve his current level of mobility.

It was then that I walked up to Steven bed space, he had the curtain drawn around him which I found suspicious. As I peered through the gap in the curtains, I looked on in shock as his wife, son, and friends carried Steven from the bed into the chair.

"Look you need to be careful with assisting Steven into the chair like that, you could cause an injury to yourself and him," I warned. "Well it's none of your flaming business what we do is up to us, so keep out of it!" shouted Stevens's aggressive wife. I quickly backed away without realising that in the corner of the room, the social worker Shirley had recorded what she observed in her folder. She walked up to me, "Don't worry Chris I will take over from here," she murmured.

Mealtimes came around and Mal became very agitated shouting that he needed a shave, His face started to boil red with anger, "I need a shave," he persisted. It was then that Sister Bridget appeared with a bowl of got water, shaving foam and a razor, "I will help you with a shave, Chris can you go to the staffroom Kate would like to speak to?"

I nervously walked into the staffroom; Kate was sitting with my final nursing grades. She showed me the grades on the paper which showed a pass grade onto all the nursing competencies. I felt such a sense of achievement that I had passed. All my work over the three-year period had amounted this.

Kate presented me with a cake which had the words 'congratulations Chris' on the icing. "Well done. you have been a great asset to the ward, and you will be a fantastic nurse!" Kate smiled. "I have to be honest with you, I was offered the part of the scarecrow for a theatre company in New York, and I have accepted the offer as it's my dream role. I just had to complete my training as a student nurse to finish my journey." I began.

"Just follow your heart, if your dream is to be an actor then go for it.

I thanked Kate, and all the staff, and took one last look onto the ward and realised how much I had changed as a person since the start of my placement.

When I started as a student nurse, I was shy and naive and had very little life experience. Now I had helped to care for people in their darkest moments, saved people's lives, looked after dying patients and their families, and helped make a difference to the wellbeing of the patients in my care. Achieving all of this, whilst losing my best friend, my brother Michael.

I lay on my bed that night, the final night before I was to fly to New York for the start of rehearsals. I lay in my bed night I couldn't sleep. I left the window open and could hear the choir of crickets in the background, as the light from the moon shone on my face. It was time for me to move on from my life and start my new beginning. Before I fell asleep, I noticed a single white feather on the window ledge. Ever since Michael passed away, I saw so many white feathers, it felt like it was his way of communicating to me, letting me know he was always listening to me.

I arrived in New York the following day and rented a two-bedroom apartment in Manhattan. Rehearsals were long and exhausting from 6am to 6pm each day, every line had to be perfect, every move and dance routine had to be perfectly synchronized in time to the music.

Rehearsals ran for over three weeks, and then it came to opening night.

I remember how nervous I was waiting behind the red curtain, the theatre auditorium was full of waiting customers, and reporters, with their camera lights flashing. There I was, standing in my scarecrow costume, as the director counted down from ten. I felt my whole-body tremble, I took a deep breath and walked onto the stage.

Chapter 11: University life

My days at university as a student nurse were just as busy as my days on placement. Many of the lectures ran over a whole day from 9-5pm. Many of the essays and exams coincided with my time on placement which made the experience just as hard.

In the first year as a student, I had to complete an essay related to the professional standards of nursing, and a practical examination. As part of the examination I had to accurately record and perform the blood pressure, heart rate, and breathing rate of a college professor, and take the manual pulse, and answer basic physiology questions.

I remember how nervous I was before entering the practical examination, waiting in a long corridor with over fifty students. We had spent time checking the pulse rate of our peers and took each other's observation in our clinical skills session. I managed to pass the exam, recording the observations accurately and answered questions relating the function of the heart and lungs.

In the second year the assessments increased in difficulty. I had to complete an once assessment. OSCE stands for objective structured clinical examination. As part of the assessment we had to interact with a mannequin, and we were giving a mews score, the total score of the clinical observation of the patient, and a description of the condition of the patient. We had to talk through how we would treat the patient based on the clinical results.

I remember walking into the examination, and the mannequin lay on the bed, in her spotty gown with big green googly eyes, and wild curly blonde hair.

I felt it very hard to interact with the mannequin, especially when the mannequin I was placed with had one hand. I went into the clinic room and greeted the mannequin explaining I would take their observation. The clinical educators explained the observational readings, and I then had to calculate the score which I completed incorrectly, the clinical educators stated she was suffering from diabetes and is at present suffering from a hypo attack. I seemed to freeze at the clinical questions, relating to the physiology by the lectures being unable to answer common medical terms I had revised.

I had failed the assessment because I did not gain consent to treat the mannequin, and I had incorrectly calculated the Mews score. I put in a lot of work to complete the reassessment and passed.

I found the practical assessments very difficult, whilst the essays including the final dissertation were a strong point of me.

The final assessment was a ten-minute presentation based on teamwork in the NHS, I had to stand up in front of twenty of my peers and two clinical educators and discuss how teamwork had been a pivotal part of my journey as a student nurse.

My time at the university was very useful, I took part in simulations to help see how patients feel when they are suffering from chronic health conditions. For example, we wore inflatable body outfits, which were specially designed to let us know what life is like living with arthritis. In one clinical session we worked with a partner, and one wore a blindfold whilst the person helped guide their partner around the university, to experience what life was like living with sight loss.

Every year as part of our course, we had to complete CPR training and manual handling training, to help us become proficient in using hoists, and with mobilising patients in the clinical environment.

At the start of my Nurse training there were twenty students in my seminar group, by the time I finished there were fifteen. Many students left for reasons such as choosing the wrong career path, having a difficult mentor, or struggling financially to stay on the course.

Chapter 12: The final wish

A year had passed since I qualified as a nurse, and I had now spent a year travelling across America in the stage show of 'the wizard of oz.' After our successful run in Broadway in New York, we travelled to California, Texas, Los Angeles and California. I rented a studio apartment in New York overlooking Manhattan. I lived the dream I always shared with Michael, to travel all over America. It felt wonderful to be performing each night in front of sell out audiences, to hear the audience clap, and to meet fans of the show after made the experience even more wonderful.

In a way working as an actor in America helped me in my grief, I was away from home, away from so many memories. Michael was with me all the time, I just needed to experience freedom, and to participate in the career of my dreams.

December came and it was time for me to make the journey home. The tour of the show would recommence in February 2016. I sat on the eleven-hour flight, reflecting on my progress of the previous year, winning an award for best stage show at the national actor's awards show, making new friends, and achieving a good income. The taxi ride home to York was filled with both fear and anticipation. I wondered what life was like since I left for my parents and Susan. I trudged through the heavy snow up to the long pathway of my family home.

It was now 6pm, and I shivered as the winter breeze brushed past me.

Our house and oak trees outside were decorated in red flashing Christmas lights. I entered the home and into the dining room, suddenly Mum Dad and Louise jumped out from behind the sofa, shouting, 'surprise' wearing party hats, and throwing confetti into the air. The living room was filled with multi coloured balloons, and banners which read 'welcome home.'

"We are so pleased to see you, we have waited so long," Mum beamed. "We have two surprises for you," Dad added. "Firstly, we want to announce that we are getting married on Boxing Day, at St Thomas Church, and the other surprise is in the red Christmas bag, under the tree." Mum smiled excitedly.

I nervously walked up to the Christmas tree, and took out the present from the red Christmas bag, it was wrapped in blue wrapping paper with a rag attached which read, 'To Chris, my 'final wish' Michael.'

I started to shake and tremble, inside was a blank DVD case with a DVD inside. "You see Chris, Michael wanted us all to watch this on Christmas as his final wish to us all, we have had to wait a year to see it, and now it's time! "Mum cried, wiping a tear from her face.

I inserted the DVD, and we all sat together on the couch. It was Michael on the DVD delivering his final hopes and wishes for us in the future. It was recorded five days before he passed away. He was sitting on his bed, with his nasal spec's oxygen mask attached to his face, he sat smiling. He explained in the video that he wanted Mum and Dad to keep talking to each other, and to visit the cottage he bought them, he advised them to go on holiday, and too give away his clothes and money to charity.

He then thanked Susan for all her help in setting up the cottage and asked her to go back to law school to achieve her dream of being a lawyer, and to not to be afraid to push herself. He then explained he found it hardest to say goodbye to me. He did not want me to let his death hold me back, he advised me to travel, make friends with strangers, travel all over America, and to know that he will always be with me. He thanked us all for the wonderful life he had, and then the camera faded to black. I began to cry, and that night as I lay in bed the

white feather lay by the window ledge.

It has now been over five years since I have completed my training. I now have worked as an actor in various stage shows in America, including the lion king, Aladdin, and the nutcracker. I still reside in New York, and my parents have recently moved to Manhattan, and we visit Louise in Devon twice a year.

My experience as student nurse changed my life, when I started my nurse training, I was an inexperienced young adult. I developed empathy and compassion, looking after dying patients holding their hands in their final moments, I have saved lives completing CPR, and I have helped improve the mental wellbeing of patients in my care. Most of all I have made a difference to people's lives, and it is a rollercoaster journey I will never forget.

Chapter 12: Tips for student nurses

The most important tip I can offer to Student nurses is to always be mindful of your own mental health. Make sure you get enough sleep each night. It is important that you always try to make sure you eat healthy foods during your breaks, and to always make sure you have a bottle of water to drink during your shift, to boost your energy during the long shift hours.

It is vital to always keep in touch with friends and family members after a difficult shift, to help boost your own morale. Visiting a family member or friend and talking through difficulties and taking over the phone can all help improve own mental wellbeing and having a strong support network is important.

Working in a hospital setting can be very stressful at times, but exercise and leisure pursuits can make a big difference to both your physical and mental wellbeing. After your shift make time for yourself, go on a long walk, listen to music in a quiet room, go to the gym, take time to see a film. Exercising and doing something you enjoy; can improve the way you feel. Also writing down a reflection of events which occurred on a difficult shift and how you would have improved what happened can also be a useful learning tool.

Keeping a written diary as a student nurse can really help as a learning log, in which you can see what skills you have gained and what skills are still outstanding. Keeping a diary is also good as a reflection, and as evidence which can support your placement document.

As a student on placement make sure you volunteer to visit different departments, such as x ray, ultrasound, a physiotherapy department, you may not have the chance to visit these as much when you are qualified nurse, and they can really help you to understand how other healthcare professionals work to support patient care.

Visiting a neonatal ward, or a local mental health service on a voluntary visit can help you meet the full exposure of nursing needs that are not related to your nursing field.

It is vital when completing your placements to undertake research and personal reading into your ward's specialism. Mentors may want to test your knowledge, and it important to understand the physiology behind patient conditions. Some placements will offer a student information pack or a reading list, please utilize this to better understand the clinical area.

If you have difficulties or conflicts in your placement setting with your placement mentor or a member of staff on placement, try to resolve all issues calmly with the ward staff/ ward manager first. If the problem is not resolved, then it important to contact your University placement team. Do not wait until the end of the placement to raise concerns about your placement I cannot

stress this enough.

In terms of revising for your nursing exams, I found producing mind maps,

spider diagrams, particularly helpful in helping to aid my memory in exams,

draw pictures of different parts of the human anatomy, for example a pictorial

diagram of the flow of blood around the heart.

Try to keep organized, if you must complete essays/exams whilst on

placement, try to plan your days off by writing a study timetable, but make

sure you give yourself adequate breaks.

It can be useful to complete bank shifts as a healthcare assistant, especially to

boost your income, but also to get a wider experience. I would advise against

completing banks shifts in your final year, as the workload and requirements

on placement are more demanding, and I would recommend putting full focus

on your course.

It is very likely as a student nurse working on the wards, that you will come across a cardiac arrest. In the event of an emergency also try to get involved, it could be grabbing the crash trolley, helping with compressions, even grabbing the drip stand, it is great practice, and a valuable learning experience. If you have experienced a cardiac arrest on placement, record what happened, to aid in your learning.

When your complete night shifts as a student nurse, make the most of these to complete your placement documentation book. Night shifts are mostly less busy than day shifts, and they can be a great way for you to read around placement conditions and improve your knowledge as a student nurse.

If you are on placement with another student nurse, try to share your experience and share your knowledge. It can be a very useful experience to help with gaps in your knowledge, and another student can help boost your morale if you are having a bad day.

If on your placement you are placed with a senior member of staff such as senior sister on the ward, try to ask if you can work with a buddy mentor along with your main mentor. Sometimes there may be times when a senior member of staff may not be able to provide a learning experience due to extra responsibilities/ meetings they attend, remember that working with other nurses in your placement area can be valuable to see how other nurses work.

As a student it can be very useful to work with nurses who specialise in certain areas, you could work with the palliative care nurse, a nurse nutritionist, a tissue viability nurse. Make the most of this opportunity to ask questions and write a reflection of what you have learnt.

Whilst learning on placement is the most valuable experience, books which refer to clinical skills can help with gaps in knowledge.

It is vital whilst on placement to make sure you take your breaks. I often enjoyed my breaks and often walked outside to get some fresh air and I felt so much more refreshed when I came back to the setting, especially after eating a delicious lunch. Missing breaks can lead to tiredness, and can be detrimental to your health, hours of work are often long you need to make sure you REST.

When on placement in a ward setting try to always involve yourself in the doctor's ward rounds. This is a vital experience as student nurse in understanding conditions and in understanding how doctors treat certain health conditions. Ask questions to the doctor, bring a notepad around with you and record any tasks the doctor requires on paper.

At times on your nursing course you may feel stressed, if this stress is affecting your practice or personal health seek medical treatment immediately, talking to your GP or going to a counselling service can really help.

It is important that you join a union such as the royal college of nursing or unison, research the unions carefully before deciding.

Try to observe and spend time with other professionals outside of the nursing field such as physiotherapists and occupational therapists, to see the work they do to help support patients in the hospital environment. Physiotherapists can also help you to understand the use of mobility aids to support your patients with their mobility.

Try to attend a multidisciplinary team where all professionals meet on the ward to discuss the patients on the ward, and discuss the background of the patient, and steps required for discharge. As you progress in your training and if you are feeling confident you could volunteer to lead a meeting to increase your confidence.

Remain assertive, although some people naturally display assertiveness, it important to make use of this as student nurse. Be assertive in knowing what your role is a student, if you feel a staff members behaviour is detrimental to your progress speak up.

As a student nurse you are in the clinical setting to learn and to progress it is vital to speak up if you are not learning.

Make family members and friends aware of times when you are on placement and are unable to attend social events. At the end of the placement plan a break away, or a day away with friends to catch up, and use it as time to relax.

Keep organized throughout your training and keep your notes you made for your anatomy and physiology exams; you will never know when you might need them in the future.

Manage your finances; this is essential over the three years of your training. Make a weekly budget of the essential things you need whilst on placement, food, travel, and toiletries etc. If you must work as a student try to arrange to work during university time, and on the weekends, working whilst on placement can be added pressure, as you are usually expected to work full time hours as a student. Some NHS trusts offer good rates of pay for the weekend for bank staff, so if you need extra cash utilise working one or two days at the weekend or as able.

Make use of your career service at your university, most career services give you a year of support after you qualify, and they can help you with interview preparation, job searches, and they can provide you with sample job applications.

Always make sure you bring back your library books on time to avoid any unnecessary fines.

During exam timetable plan your time very carefully, but also make sure that you get over eight hours of sleep each day.

Learn common medications quickly, knowing their uses, side effects etc. As part of your nurse training you need to learn the names and uses of a wide range of medicines. Try to create a fact file of common medicines, when you are on your first placement record the medications you have come across, you may need to know their uses in the future.

A difficult skill in healthcare is trying to break bad news if you can observe the way doctors or other nurse's deliver this, it could help form your future practice.

Make sure you gain advice you need in your training from your personal tutor and nursing lecturers, they are employed to help, and will have spent a significant amount of time on the wards and will have a wealth of useful information.

Always try to point out poor practice to other members of staff, for example if staff ask to move a patient without a slide sheet, or try to mobilise a patient in an 'alternative' way, always follow the rules and regulations of your trust, poor practices or 'lazy' alternatives to help patients are negative forms of patient care.

Use wash and dressing assessments as an essential method to get to know your patient. With wash and dressing assessments you can check your patients' skin, complete a history taking assessment, assess the patient's mobility, and most importantly build a rapport with your patient, getting to know them, and letting them see what an innovative student you are.

When you are starting a placement and are orienting yourself on the ward, make a note of all the wards routines and timings of when certain clinical skills occur this will help you in the future.

Make use of the nursing handover and research any terminology or new language you come across, underline key words and conditions, later you can come back and research this. Keep a record each day on a separate piece of paper of tasks you have completed, for your handover. Try to be involved in handing over your patients in conjunction with your mentor; it is excellent practice to start this early in your training.

Thank you for reading my book. If you enjoyed it, please leave a review!

For updates follow me on Instagram @buttinchris

Good luck to any student nurses reading this on their own journey, I hope one day you can share your journey!

Printed in Great Britain
by Amazon

51218648R00128